UNDERSTANDING CHRONIC FATIGUE SYNDROME

Dr Alastair Jackson grew up and was educated in Melbourne, Australia. His interests at school included music, literature, debating and languages.

He studied Medicine at the University of Melbourne, graduating in 1973. He obtained a postgraduate degree in obstetrics four years later, but by that time had already chosen general practice as his preferred field of medicine.

In 1995, after twenty years of a very happy and fulfilling career, Dr Jackson became ill with what was initially feared to be multiple sclerosis. After many tests and several specialist opinions he was diagnosed as having chronic fatigue syndrome—a condition about which he and many others in the medical profession knew very little.

His retirement from medicine and subsequent convalescence forced him to give up many aspects of his previously active lifestyle. However, with perseverance, tolerance and adjustment he learned to cope with his illness and found his interest in its aetiology was stimulated. As he continued to improve clinically, he was able to do research into CFS and was encouraged to put his thoughts into print.

Several years later Alastair Jackson has virtually recovered from CFS. He has modified many aspects of his life and no longer practises full-time medicine. But he has occupied his time with many other interests and community activities. He enjoys music, theatre and fine arts. He is well-known as a broadcaster of opera and classical music on radio 3MBS-FM, is a director of the Melba Conservatorium of Music and is the Chairman of Opera Foundation Victoria.

UNDERSTANDING CHRONIC FATIGUE SYNDROME

Better ways of managing your lifestyle

Dr Alastair Jackson

ALLEN & UNWIN

First published in 2000

Allen & Unwin
83 Alexander Street
Crows Nest NSW 2065
Australia
Phone: (61 2) 8425 0100
Fax: (61 2) 9906 2218
E-mail: frontdesk@allen-unwin.com.au
Web: http://www.allenandunwin.com

National Library of Australia
Cataloguing-in-Publication entry:

Jackson, Alastair, 1947– .
    Understanding chronic fatigue syndrome: better ways of managing
    your lifestyle.

    Bibliography.
    Includes index.
    ISBN 1 86508 407 7.

    1. Chronic fatigue syndrome. 2. Chronic fatigue syndrome—
    Australia. I. Title.

616.0478

Illustrated by Richard Dell
Printed and bound by Australian Print Group, Maryborough, Vic.

10 9 8 7 6 5 4 3 2

Contents

Preface

It was not without some trepidation that I agreed to write this book. After all, it required a certain amount of energy, which was the one commodity I lacked. One year had elapsed since I had been forced by this illness to give up a career I loved and to become a full-time patient. But, surprisingly, I found it somewhat therapeutic to put my story into words. If it helped others to cope with a generally misunderstood condition, then the effort would be truly worth it. My mind went back to the beginning.

In late 1994 I combined a holiday break with a medical conference in sunny Queensland—one of those affairs which is half work and half play, with morning lectures and afternoons free to swim, play or simply sit around the pool and enjoy the climate.

Winter in Melbourne had brought its usual share of coughs, colds and influenza, which form a large part of the general practitioner's workload. Like most GPs, I had come into contact with a host of different viruses on a daily basis. Every winter, for as long as I could remember, I had suffered a minor upper respiratory infection, which would last a couple of days, then leave me symptom-free for the rest of the season. I believed that it probably built up my immunity and there was no reason to think 1994 would be different.

For some months prior to my holiday break I had felt tired. Even my usually relaxing sessions at the piano seemed to exhaust me. For the first time in my life playing the piano had become an effort. Probably the result of a busy year, I thought, and nothing a break wouldn't fix. I was glad it was not the overseas conference I had originally planned to attend, because I lacked the energy that would entail.

Until this time, keeping fit had been an important part of my life. Although never a sportsman, I enjoyed walking and never swam without doing a reasonable number of laps. Indeed, aerobics had been a daily routine for years, as I had a history of coronary artery disease on one side of the family. My father, who was an extremely fit and active businessman, had died suddenly of a heart attack at the age of 47—when I was eleven years old. Ironically I had just turned 47 myself and, needless to say, watched my diet and never smoked.

In fact, my lifestyle was always healthy. I tried to practise what I preached to my patients. Apart from the odd indulgence, a sweet tooth and an enjoyment of wine (now proven medically beneficial) I had never abused my body. The waistline, if it erred a little, could always be brought under control and my weight had been acceptable (and fairly constant) for many years.

Although my father died prematurely, my mother's genes were good. An indefatigable octagenerian, she has always been a tireless supporter of worthwhile causes (which included her four sons!). We spoke daily on the phone and she saw me several times each week. It was not long before she astutely noticed my depleted energy levels. Her concern confirmed what I myself had suspected. My health was below par and not improving.

The decline in my strength became even more apparent on holiday, particularly the physical exhaustion that inevitably followed what to most people would be minimal exertion. Simple walks along the beach should have been pleasurable but instead became a burden. Previously a brisk walker, I found myself needing to stop frequently. The limbs were heavy, the muscles hurt and, for the first time in my life, I thought that age must be catching up with me. And yet, I was only in my late forties. Many active people around me were much older. Many of my patients were fit and healthy 'senior citizens'. These days lots of people remain energetic achievers well into their eighties, while here was I, feeling washed up and totally drained.

Could the symptoms be those of a viral illness? There was no fever or sore throat, no cough or earache. Not even my long-term hayfever was a problem, just a muscle soreness, joint pains and total exhaustion. My appetite was fine, and my concentration and memory were not affected at this stage. But one other symptom did bother me: intermittent bilateral frontal headache, sometimes accompanied by a throbbing sensation in one eye. Fortunately all these symptoms were relieved by a combination of paracetamol, codeine and rest.

I was glad to return home—the best place to be when one is not well. I knew I needed a thorough examination and tests. The symptoms had neither worsened nor subsided. At this point they were being held in check.

Historically, doctors have not always been good patients. Some have even made the mistake of self-diagnosis, which is tempting fate. The large number of possible diagnoses spinning through my head made me feel worse. Was it multiple sclerosis, perhaps a tumour?—the list went on and on. I made an appointment to see a general practitioner whom I knew I could trust and whose advice I would respect.

By the time of my first appointment there had been some additional symptoms. Unsteadiness on descending a staircase became quite marked. For the first time ever I needed to hold the rail and walk slowly. This persisted regardless of whether my muscles were aching. Bright light also seemed to be a problem, necessitating the regular use of sunglasses. I thought the photophobia (intolerance to light) may be linked to the headaches, which felt vascular or migrainous. However, at that stage the various symptoms didn't add up.

Sleep disturbance was my other big concern. I had always been a person who could get by on five or six hours' sleep a night. This stemmed from study at university and irregular hours as a hospital resident. Regardless of when I went to bed I seldom fell asleep before midnight, and I was usually up and about by seven in the morning. But now I took even longer to get to sleep, sometimes woke through the night and always felt totally exhausted in the morning.

In my reversed role of patient I tried to remain detached and objective. The possibility of chronic fatigue syndrome (CFS) had gone through my mind, but I seriously thought my symptoms were too severe for that. Multiple sclerosis or an early malignancy seemed more likely contenders. There had been a few cases of CFS among my patients, but most had been of the post-glandular fever type. With several months of rest these patients usually improved. My condition, however, was worsening by the month and I needed to know why.

A thorough history was taken, followed by a complete physical examination. To my relief there were no signs of enlarged glands or liver. A neurological assessment revealed no major discrepancy and the only abnormal finding was a blood pressure reading somewhat higher than normal. My anxiety probably accounted for that!

Routine tests were ordered. These included full blood count, erythrocyte sedimentation rate, thyroid screen and various blood tests to exclude liver, renal and rheumatoid illness. My urine was examined, my chest X-rayed and a brain scan ordered.

At my next appointment the results were discussed. My symptoms had not changed and I had, by this time, become rather depressed. In a way I wished something definite *had* been found to explain the way I felt. My GP was understanding and noted every symptom. Her view was that CFS was a very likely diagnosis, but she wanted a second opinion.

In the meantime, on her advice, I had curtailed my work-load. Over a period of almost twenty years I had built up my share of a very busy practice in the inner suburban Melbourne district of Toorak. Unlike many recent clinics, which rely on locum services, the practice provided 24-hour cover, which was of obvious advantage to patients but unquestionably demanding of doctors. Now I felt that I was not able to give more than one session a day, starting later and with patient numbers strictly controlled. This was a compromise I was prepared to make if it meant a quicker recovery. With a considerably shortened working day I was able to cope, but knew that my limited reserves were being used to the full.

My specialist covered my symptoms in even greater detail. His examination revealed no major abnormality and he was happy with the pathology results. He confirmed the diagnosis and talked at length of its implications. He agreed that I should continue as I was, provided the symptoms got no worse. And I was relieved at last to have a diagnosis with which two doctors in whom I had the greatest confidence had concurred.

My appointments continued on a regular basis—initially fortnightly, then monthly, with both my doctors. With each visit I felt the fear of the unknown subsiding, and my confidence was at last starting to return.

As there was no specific cure we discussed management of the illness at great length. I had been advised to take non-steroidal anti-inflammatory drugs on a regular dosage to reduce the myalgia (muscle pain), with the addition of hot pads, daily hydrotherapy and bed rest when needed. Painkillers were an optional extra, which I certainly needed from time to time.

The other medication prescribed was an antidepressant. I had frankly become depressed with the changes that had occurred. The alteration of my lifestyle and the limits imposed upon me by CFS were enough to make me so. But to this day I am sure, as are my doctors, that the depression was *not* a part of my initial illness. Instead, it was a secondary symptom—a reaction to what had happened. For that reason I commenced a nightly dose of antidepressant medication for the first time in my life. I believe it helped me to cope with the physical symptoms, which were, at their worst, quite devastating.

Despite a conservative nature, I was interested to learn of every alternative therapy suggested for CFS. I have always kept an open mind on all things medical and was curious to know what was being considered as a possible treatment. But I was also not so naive as to believe that some of the treatments suggested could do any good at all. My specialist had told me early on not to be tempted, no matter how frustrated I became, by alternative remedies. His valuable advice was to treat the symptoms, not look for a magical cure. So, apart from the prescribed medication, the only other treatment I had at this stage were regular injections of gamma-globulin and intramuscular B-group vitamins from my GP. They left me feeling slightly better, but in retrospect her understanding and compassion probably played a more significant role.

Another great help during this period was a book by the English medical doctor, Charles Shepherd (*Living With M.E.*). Like me, he had been in general practice but had been forced into retirement by CFS, with which he had struggled for over a decade. His book answered a lot of my questions and helped me to adjust my lifestyle. His thorough treatment of the condition and his optimism in adversity were ideal adjuncts to the treatment I was already receiving.

The sleep disturbances improved a little. They were quite obviously a symptom of the depression that had occurred as a result of the CFS. That they responded to antidepressant treatment supports this. And that the medication did nothing to help the physical symptoms (myalgia, etc.) was also an indication that depression tends to be a consequence, rather than a primary symptom, of CFS.

The summer months rolled on as I continued on a level 'plateau'. I lived one day at a time, seeing patients for three hours and conserving my limited energy for the remainder of the day. Friends and family were of great emotional support, as were most of the patients. I can think of only a few who implied that 'doctors have no right to be ill'.

By March 1995 I had been on treatment for four months. I had learned to manage my life as best I could. Help was accepted when necessary, although I tried to be as independent as possible. My day started slowly and followed a routine. Mild stretching exercises in a warm bath led to gradual mobilisation.

Days became categorised as simply 'good' or 'bad'. The exhaustion was always present to some degree. If the muscle fatigue did not turn to pain, and if I was able to accomplish a few minor tasks, then the day was good. A bad day meant most of the time was spent in bed with painkillers in addition to the routine medication.

Some of the days were totally unpredictable. The myalgia would be constant without any significant exertion at all. It took some time to realise that the symptoms could be delayed up to 24 hours. I sometimes thought I had been able to perform a task without pain, only to be reminded the next day that I had been foolish to try.

By May the symptoms were becoming more severe. One particularly bad weekend was spent entirely in bed. It was at that time that I realised that even part-time work would have to cease. It had become a matter of priorities. Above all else I desperately wanted to get over this condition and to give my body a chance to recover totally. My career had to be put on hold. We have only one chance at life, and I could feel mine slipping away.

The months that followed brought a slow improvement. It took me a long time to get used to the erratic pattern of remissions and relapses. But, with time, I could feel myself moving from one plateau to another. 'Good' days outnumbered 'bad', and at last I felt recovery was within reach.

By the end of 1996 I still felt my days were effectively shortened. The number of available useful hours was reduced. But the quality of those useful hours improved and I was approaching normality for a larger part of each day.

The next twelve months saw my CFS in 'stable plateau' mode, with occasional dips. Sometimes my own activities caused a temporary relapse for which I had only myself to blame. This remained the most difficult aspect of managing CFS.

By 1998 I felt vastly improved. The number and severity of relapses were greatly reduced and my ability to perform normal physical tasks was almost back to what it had been prior to the onset of CFS. The progress since then has continued. I am now involved in a wide range of interests and community activities, but they are taken at my own pace. I have adapted my lifestyle accordingly and feel that this, in fact, has actually been a benefit of having had CFS.

Whether you are a sufferer of CFS or a friend or relative of one, may this book be a help and a guide to coping. Above all, may it be a reassurance that things really can improve. As with many other illnesses, I cannot emphasise enough the importance of optimism. Time is often the best healer, and most CFS patients improve substantially, with many making a complete recovery. During that time it is necessary to manage the condition and cope with the symptoms as best you can. If my book can help other CFS sufferers to achieve this, then I will feel it has been worthwhile.

Alastair Jackson
August 2000

What is chronic fatigue syndrome (CFS)?

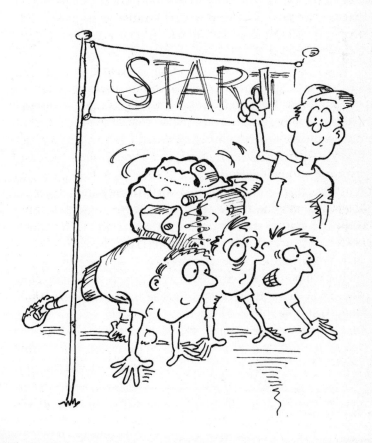

In recent years few illnesses have been less understood than chronic fatigue syndrome (CFS), also known as 'myalgic encephalomyelitis' (ME). By its very name there has been a tendency to trivialise it. Everyone suffers fatigue, some more than others; but few realise that overwhelming fatigue is just one part of the multi-faceted syndrome that makes up CFS.

Myalgic encephalomyelitis is not accurate terminology either. It implies an inflammation of the brain and spinal cord which is rare, severe and often fatal. But there is involvement of the brain ('encephalo'), the nervous system ('myelo') and the muscles ('myalgia' is muscle pain). The degree to which the muscles, brain and nervous system are affected will vary between patients and also fluctuate in frequency and severity within the same patient, even from one day to the next. A better term would be 'myalgic encephalopathy'.

The major symptom of the condition is a constant feeling of tiredness. Anyone who has had a bad case of influenza or glandular fever will know how severe the associated fatigue can be. Imagine the devastation of that situation persisting for many months or, more commonly, for several years. That it is exacerbated by even the mildest physical exertion makes it even worse. The simplest of tasks becomes a major effort and may well result in increasing severity of the muscle fatigue, to the point where it becomes painful.

In addition to the muscular fatigue or pain, CFS patients suffer an array of associated symptoms. These are usually attributed to the cerebral component of the illness, and include memory impairment, difficulty in concentration, disturbed sleep patterns and muscle incoordination which makes simple physical tasks a great challenge. Neural (nerve) involvement may cause paraesthesia (disturbed sense of touch or numbness) and altered proprioception (sense of position), which in turn can result in balance disturbance, especially when walking up or down stairs. Headaches are a frequent symptom, with visual and speech disturbances noted in some patients.

Allergies and infections can also be a problem in some patients. Possibly through immune dysfunction, some patients report increased susceptibility to sore throats, yeast and fungal infections, allergies or hypersensitivities, and lymph node enlargement. These tend to be more apparent in the early stages of the illness but may recur in certain cases.

The very nature of the symptoms restricts one's lifestyle and activities. The effective number of useful hours in a day is often halved, even when the patient is in a stable or plateau phase of the illness. Running on half-charged or run-down batteries is a common description of how many CFS patients feel, especially in the first twelve months of the illness. With trial and error and the passage of time they learn to ration their limited energy reserves. Proper management of the condition will ensure that they recognise their limitations.

Needless to say, depression is also an inevitable consequence of CFS. But, contrary to some views, it is not usually a primary symptom. Anybody having to alter their lifestyle, possibly cease working and find their activities heavily curtailed, is naturally going to be depressed. Spending many months almost bed-bound is hardly likely to improve one's psyche. Antidepressants may sometimes be useful, but in many cases they have no major effect on the syndrome or its course.

The exact aetiology (cause) of CFS is unknown. Various research groups believe a virus to be the most likely cause, coupled with an abnormal immune response. This may be due to persistent viral infection or an overreaction or prolonged response of the patient's immune system. The resultant build-up of chemical 'messengers' within the immune system is then thought to create the symptoms that characterise CFS.

Other postulated causes include the effect of a persistent virus on various sections of the brain, although this has not been established and has been refuted by some researchers. Abnormalities in cerebral perfusion (blood flow) and disturbed function of the hypothalamic and pituitary sections of the brain are thought to disturb hormone and neurotransmitter production in CFS patients. Low total body potassium and the effect of pesticides have also been implicated.

As yet there is no laboratory test to diagnose CFS. Diagnosis is made on the basis of the patient's history and symptoms and on the exclusion of other conditions. It is imperative that certain baseline tests be performed, including blood and urine pathology screens. Specific markers have been found in the urine of CFS patients, which may eventually result in a test for the condition.

There is no specific treatment for CFS. Management is mostly directed at symptomatic relief and modification of lifestyle. Certain therapies have proved beneficial in some sufferers, but most have no scientific basis, while a few may actually be harmful. Medications may help certain aspects of the illness such as muscle pain, sleep disturbances and allergies. Most effective are common sense measures such as rest when necessary and the avoidance of aggravating factors.

Support from doctors is crucial. Their knowledge about the condition can increase patients' feeling of confidence and control. Understanding from family and friends of the limitations imposed by CFS is vital to patients' well-being, as is the empathy of employers, schools and others in the general community.

In Australia and New Zealand, the United Kingdom and the USA, the establishment of CFS support groups has been of great importance. They have helped increase community awareness and have offered patients active involvement through regular newsletters and meetings. They have encouraged the participation of doctors and health workers and have been instrumental in the ongoing research into CFS and its management. (A range of international support organisations are listed following Chapter 7.)

The latter half of the twentieth century has seen enormous advances in medical science and knowledge. The development of ultrasound, scanning, laser and digital technologies has revolutionised the diagnoses, prevention and treatment of so many diseases. Medicine itself has become super specialised, with new fields and more puzzles to solve. And yet some basic mysteries remain. The cure for the common cold is as evasive as ever. On a more serious level, understanding the exact nature of the HIV virus and the possibility of developing a vaccine remain huge challenges—as do cures for many cancers and other chronic illnesses.

CFS is such a condition. Though not a new illness, it is receiving more attention and being diagnosed more often today than decades ago, when it was shrouded in mystery. But there is a clear need for ongoing research to give insight into its pathophysiology and guidance as to its management. Despite our limited knowledge and treatment options, it is up to the medical profession to recognise the disorder and to educate and support affected patients. Certain elements of CFS management could apply equally well to other chronic conditions, and I will enlarge upon this where appropriate.

There is nothing new about CFS. As with many other illnesses, there is evidence to suggest that it has been around for centuries. The fact that more has been written about it in recent years is due to the illness being recognised more for what it is—a seriously disabling and chronic disorder that is, at last, being taken seriously by the medical profession.

As long ago as the mid-eighteenth century, medical literature recorded a disorder characterised by profound fatigue and associated physical symptoms with little or no clinical abnormalities. For years Florence Nightingale suffered a mystery illness that featured many of the symptoms of CFS. That she managed to establish the first formal school of nursing and founded the International Red Cross was quite remarkable, but fits with the image of many CFS sufferers being achievers. Evolutionist Charles Darwin was another renowned figure who had an undiagnosed debilitating illness that resembled CFS in many ways.

The medical profession remained indifferent to the subject until the mid-1930s in the USA. It was in Los Angeles in 1934 that a localised outbreak of a viral-type illness was noted. It involved, ironically, doctors and nurses working at the Los Angeles County General Hospital. Symptoms of a flu-type illness were followed by severe fatigue and muscle weakness. Poliomyelitis was at first considered, until the absence of muscle wasting ruled out that diagnosis. Most recovered over a period of time, although many were affected for more than six months.

It was not until half a century later that Americans really became aware of the condition. In 1985, at Lake Tahoe in Nevada, an outbreak of a similar mystery illness occurred. Previously fit adults in their thirties and forties reported a flu-like illness, which was then followed by muscular fatigue and neuropsychiatric dysfunction involving concentration and short-term memory. Almost all were successful and active high achievers, with many professionals among them. Thus the term 'yuppie flu' originated, and the magazine *Newsweek* referred to it as the 'malaise of the Eighties'. The fact that pathology tests were normal gave rise to doubt about the authenticity of the disease. And yet, the group of people most affected were the last type to stay away from work without good reason. The symptoms were real enough, and many of the patients presented initially with sore throats, glandular enlargement and low-grade fever.

The outbreak attracted the interest of two dedicated doctors, Dan Peterson and Paul Cheney. They had no doubt that these patients were genuinely ill. The similarity of their symptoms to glandular fever made them wonder about a viral aetiology. In particular they suspected the Epstein-Barr virus (EBV), which causes glandular fever or infectious mononucleosis. As with many viruses, the EBV remains in the body after infection. The healthy person's immune system usually produces antibodies to such a virus and bestows lifetime immunity.

The doctors proposed that an abnormal immune

response may be involved. Something was allowing the dormant virus to become reactivated. With multiplication of the virus and an inadequate immune system there followed a recurrent, persisting infection which would produce chronic symptoms. It was known that the Epstein-Barr virus belonged to the herpes group and that members of the herpes group, such as the cold sore virus, could be reactivated at times of stress or when the immune system was compromised in some way.

The Lake Tahoe patients were tested for EBV. Raised antibodies to EBV were found in about 75 per cent of them, but some had normal levels and a few had no antibodies at all. A similar result could be expected in a control (or normal) group, so the results were inconclusive.

The Lake Tahoe outbreak eventually subsided. It had stimulated interest in the possible role of a virus at the very time that the AIDS epidemic was capturing headlines around the world. The resultant research is ongoing and will undoubtedly benefit the treatment of all viral illnesses as we enter the twenty-first century.

Following the occurrence of a CFS-type illness in Los Angeles in 1934, a similar syndrome was reported in many other parts of the world including Europe, South Africa, Australia and, most famously, the United Kingdom. All cases had symptoms which came within the same spectrum, with minor variations. And each outbreak attracted attention due to the large number of patients involved, even though sporadic individual cases were always presenting.

The widespread occurrence in so many different countries resulted in a multiplicity of names for the syndrome. Only in recent years has the term 'chronic fatigue syndrome'— although far from ideal—been universally recognised.

Outbreaks were documented in Switzerland, Greece, Denmark and Iceland. The 1948 Iceland epidemic involved over a thousand cases, mostly high school students. Interestingly, when a polio epidemic swept Iceland seven years later, those who had previously been afflicted with the

CFS-type illness (termed 'Icelandic disease') were immune to the polio. This suggested that the original infection had produced, like a vaccination, a degree of immunity. The implication of a similar virus was very strong, although it was never isolated.

A major epidemic occurred in Adelaide, Australia in 1949, preceded by a polio epidemic several months earlier. The CFS-type cases continued until 1951 by which time there were nearly 700 hospital admissions. No virus was ever identified. A similar occurrence in New Zealand resulted in the syndrome being labelled 'Tapanui flu'. In early 1955 a major outbreak occurred in Durban, South Africa. As in Iceland and Australia, it coincided with a polio epidemic. Most of those affected in Durban were nursing and medical staff. The symptoms were identical to those cases previously identified elsewhere.

Perhaps the best documented of outbreaks was that at the Royal Free Hospital in London in July 1955. Patients were admitted with typical respiratory symptoms—sore throat, enlarged lymph glands and a low-grade fever. Some developed dizziness, headaches and paraesthesia (abnormal skin sensations), and all of them had disturbances of concentration and short-term memory. However, the most striking feature of their illness was profound muscle fatigue brought on by minimal physical exertion. Like previous outbreaks in the USA, Iceland and Australia, the symptoms were at first suggestive of polio, still a threat in those pre-vaccination days. However, no muscle wasting became evident and other investigations proved normal. The illness ran a similar course to those cases reported previously.

The 'Royal Free disease', as it was called, went on to involve almost 300 patients. The hospital's own medical and nursing staff were not immune, and so many were taken ill that the hospital was forced to close for several months. The pattern of symptoms was characteristic: an initial flu-like illness was followed by neuromuscular involvement, cerebral disturbance and profound muscular fatigue. The term 'myalgic encephalopathy' was first used in an article published in the *Lancet* medical journal a year later by Dr Melvin Ramsay, consultant physician at the Royal Free Hospital at the time of the outbreak.

The outbreaks described above have been the most-documented occurrences of CFS. They are by no means the only ones, with many less spectacular episodes occurring over the last few decades. And although I have referred to 'outbreaks' it should be emphasised that CFS is not contagious in the normal sense of the word. Rather it is 'endemic', with individual cases occurring all the time. Although a viral infection can spread easily from person to person, susceptibility to a persistence of that infection and to its becoming CFS is not something that is passed on. The documented outbreaks have tended to occur in closed communities such as schools (Iceland, 1948) or hospitals (Los Angeles, 1934; London, 1955).

Although exact figures are not available, it would appear that the majority of patients with CFS make a complete recovery or improve significantly within a five-year period. Some will follow a pattern of remission alternating with relapse, while a minority remain chronically unwell.

No two patients with CFS are affected in quite the same way. The individual nature of the illness makes it important that no-one should give up hope of a permanent recovery, regardless of how bad the initial symptoms may be. Obviously, the earlier the correct diagnosis is made the sooner the illness will be managed appropriately. A good prognosis is more likely as a result.

With a greater understanding of CFS the prognosis can only improve. Although we have a number of theories regarding its aetiology, the disorder has a certain amount in common with other entero-viral illnesses (the group to which the polio virus belongs). There are also implications regarding the immune system and the body's ability to cope with stress. This book will examine the best ways of managing CFS with the aim of effecting a complete recovery.

Chapter two

Aetiology—What causes CFS?

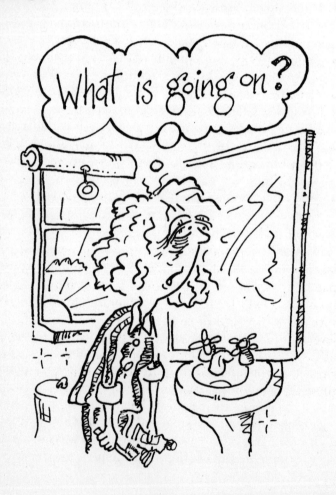

The results of major studies in recent years have thrown light on both the epidemiology (prevalence and distribution in the community) and aetiology (cause) of chronic fatigue syndrome. Although some progress has been made we are still far from understanding the exact nature of the illness. But some things are known:

- CFS appears to be triggered by an acute viral illness in many cases. The remainder have a more insidious onset (still probably infectious). Other possible 'trigger factors' are discussed below.
- Peak onset is between the age of 20 and 40 years, but sufferers can be as young as five years and the illness can present for the first time in a patient over 70 years.
- Incidence in the community appears to be 0.1 per cent to 0.2 per cent of the general population.
- More females are affected, the female:male ratio being approximately 2:1. However, women are more likely to present earlier and are considered more at risk.
- The socio-economic profile of CFS patients is similar to that of the population as a whole. 'Yuppie flu' is a total misnomer.
- There are no obvious differences with regard to race, although it has been studied more in the developed nations.

The study of the mechanism of symptom production has led researchers to discover certain abnormalities in CFS patients. The implications of these findings have suggested possible causes. These include immune abnormalities, disturbance in blood flow to parts of the brain and increased levels of certain enzymes in the blood—all of which can affect neuromuscular function. These are presumably caused by an infection (usually viral), with possibly the presence of one or more other 'trigger factors'.

Trigger factors that can help a virus to stimulate an abnormal immune response

Genetic risk factors

A defective immune response to a viral (or other) infection may be inherited. CFS has been noted to affect first-degree relatives living apart, suggesting some hereditary factor may be involved. Likewise, the genetic link in some forms of arthritis and certain malignancies has been known for years. Research with common genetic markers (called HLA antigens) is ongoing.

Recent research has also revealed that a virus may be activated when a person's metabolism is altered due to increased levels of fatty acids. The fatty acid level appears to be influenced by genetic factors.

Allergies or hypersensitivities

The immune system is an integral part of the allergic response. The level of IgE antibodies is raised in patients who are having an allergic reaction. Interestingly, many CFS patients have noticed less allergy-type symptoms during the course of their illness. Sometimes the return of troublesome allergic rhinitis (hay fever), pruritus or asthma may actually correspond with a remission of their CFS symptoms.

Others have reported a flare-up of allergic symptoms, whether or not there was a pre-existing allergy. The effects of a persisting virus and/or the continuation of a low-grade immune response may 'unmask' an allergy in a susceptible individual.

However, it should be remembered that allergies are extremely common in the general community. And the nature of an allergy can change at different stages of a patient's life. So the allergic 'trigger', although relevant in some CFS patients, is by no means common to all cases. As I will stress later in the book, the existence of CFS does not preclude other medical problems. It is sometimes easy to blame all manner of symptoms on a particular diagnosis without strong evidence.

Physical or mental stress

Like so many illnesses, CFS is aggravated by stress. Stress may be a co-factor in increasing your susceptibility at the time of the initial infection. Stress may be:

i *physical:* Athletes training strenuously are known to have an altered immune response. And the link between vigorous exertion and the complications of an enteroviral infection (e.g. Coxsackie endocarditis) can be life-threatening.

Any acute infection, together with vigorous training and stress (both physical and emotional), are co-factors that may precipitate CFS in certain individuals. Studies in Melbourne have shown that 78 per cent of athletes who develop CFS experience an acute onset of the illness, with the remainder reporting a gradual decline in health.

ii *mental:* Major family crises, bereavements, operations, employment changes and other important 'life events' can impair the immune response to infection. Such stresses can also affect the way people cope with illness. This important aspect of managing CFS will be dealt with in greater detail later in the book.

Exposure to chemicals and pesticides

As society becomes more 'sophisticated' and the 'rat race' progresses, we can become more reliant on man-made diversions and short cuts to a more streamlined lifestyle. We lean towards fast foods, jet travel, smoggy cities, cigarettes and alcohol. There is no doubt that our immune responses will be adversely affected as a result. The body cannot cope with continuing environmental pollution, which strains and overloads our individual immune systems. Chapter 5 discusses the importance of diet and lifestyle in treating not only CFS but also other chronic illnesses. Preventive medicine is more important now than ever as we enter the twenty-first century.

Research from the University of Newcastle in Australia has confirmed the presence of elevated levels of organochlorine pesticides in some CFS patients. In fact, the number of CFS patients with elevated levels of hexachlorobenzene was more than twice that of a healthy control group, which is statistically significant. But because such levels can be found in healthy individuals, larger epidemiological studies are required and stringent criteria would need to be satisfied before a causal link could be confirmed.

Neurally mediated hypotension

Recent studies in the USA have indicated an association between CFS and neurally mediated hypotension (NMH). NMH is also known as 'vasodepressor syncope' or 'neurocardiogenic syncope' and involves an abnormal reflex between heart and brain. It's a form of low blood pressure that occurs after a prolonged period of standing, but differs from the more common 'orthostatic' hypotension. The symptoms include light-headedness, abdominal discomfort, blurred vision and pallor. The prolonged fatigue after syncope (fainting) is prominent. Part of the therapy is to increase both salt and fluid intake. These measures are discussed in more detail in Chapter 6.

Let us look in more detail at the postulated causes of CFS.

Conditions likely to cause CFS

Immunological abnormalities

Although the exact cause of CFS is unknown, many leading researchers in Australia, the United Kingdom and the USA believe that the symptoms are produced by a continuing abnormal immune response. This may be due to:

- a persisting infection or several infections at once
- the failure of the immune response to 'turn off' after an initial infection
- an inappropriate response or 'overreaction' by the immune system to an immune challenge, e.g. viral or bacterial infections, vaccinations.

The end result is the production of an excessive amount of cytokines, which have the role of chemical messengers of the immune system. They travel freely in the body, and their effect on neural (nerve) and muscular tissues is to produce the symptoms that characterise CFS.

The immune system has the role of recognising and removing potentially harmful invader micro-organisms from the body. In the case of CFS, the invading micro-organism has been presumed to be viral. The initial clinical symptoms are often viral in type. And despite the fact that no single virus has ever been identified, the general feeling among research scientists is that a virus is involved in many cases, at least in the initial stages of CFS. It may even be a long-standing latent virus that has been reactivated by a certain 'trigger' factor (see above).

The immune system is stimulated by special white blood cells called 'T4 helper lymphocytes'. They recognise the virus as an invader and set about producing cytokines. These cytokines act like messenger chemicals and their build-up in brain, nerve and muscle tissue accounts for some of the symptoms of CFS or, indeed, any acute viral infection. The cytokines also encourage the immune reaction by increasing the production of antibodies. These are proteins, or immunoglobulins, derived from plasma cells, which originate in the bone marrow. They attach to the viral particles and make them susceptible to attack by the macrophages (or 'scavenger' cells).

Any condition affecting the bone marrow will damage the body's ability to produce plasma cells and thus anti-bodies. In diseases like leukaemia, bone marrow transplants have been carried out where the leukaemia cells infiltrated the bone marrow.

Different types of antibodies are produced following a viral infection. IgA antibodies, the first type, are manufactured by regional lymph glands, which enlarge as a result. In the acute situation, IgA antibodies prevent blood spread of the virus, but they are not long-lasting.

IgG and IgM antibodies are then manufactured and may remain indefinitely in the blood. They are specific to a particular virus, and their production is stimulated by vaccination, often leading to lifelong protection from that particular virus.

The immune response is normally slowed down when the infection is under control. This is the job of the T8 suppressor lymphocytes. Any deficiency of these white blood cells would see a continuing immune reaction. The energy needed to produce more cytokines, more antibodies and more macrophage activity would soon deplete a patient's energy reserves. The constant cellular activity, or 'immune overdrive' could well explain the fatigue component of CFS.

Any abnormal ratio of T4 helper and T8 suppressor lymphocyte cells would throw one's immune system out of kilter. This aspect of abnormal immune response has attracted the attention of many researchers who, unfortunately, have not always produced consistent findings.

Unlike AIDS (acquired immune deficiency syndrome) from HIV (human immunodeficiency virus), the abnormalities with the T4 and T8 lymphocyte numbers in CFS are not characteristic. Despite subtle changes in certain parameters there is no specific abnormality with the lymphocytes that could be considered diagnostic. Most of the findings are more consistent with a persisting viral infection than an immunodeficiency disorder.

Despite the lack of specificity there is no doubt the immune system is involved. There is ongoing research to try to identify an excess or deficiency of chemicals or enzymes that have a direct or indirect effect on immune function.

Immunology is a fascinating but exacting science. Its complexities go far beyond the scope of this book. Suffice to say that the immune system holds the answer to many of the mysteries of CFS and, indeed, many other medical conditions including cancer and autoimmune disease. At each international CFS conference many of the papers deal with the findings of medical scientists who have measured different immunological parameters. Their research tries to find a logical connection between abnormalities demonstrated in the laboratory and the various clinical facets of chronic fatigue.

Some of the findings in recent years have suggested (but not proven) that:

- CFS is a persistent viral illness despite the fact that no specific virus has been identified
- CFS may, in fact, be two separate diseases—one with a gradual onset (perhaps endocrine or hormone related), and another with an acute onset (of presumably infectious nature)
- the absence in CFS patients of a 'suppressor' cytokine would explain the immune reaction's failure to turn off in this condition
- certain cytokines which produce the symptoms of CFS may be reduced through treatment with vitamin E and other anti-oxidants
- although the female:male ratio in CFS is 2:1, females are surprisingly more resistant to infection than males because of an increased sensitivity of the immune system—it is more on guard; however it is because of this that females are more susceptible to autoimmune disease, where the immune system attacks cells of the body as if they were foreign invaders.

Too many uncertainties exist for a consensus to be reached at this time. It makes sense that the most cost-effective immunological parameters are measured in CFS research studies.

The standardisation of testing is also important. Serum samples vary widely according to collection materials, storage conditions and temperature control. Cytokines are very sensitive to freezing and thawing, and how the serum is handled can affect results.

It is also interesting that only 20–40 per cent of the CFS population has any single immune problem at a given moment. For this reason it may make sense to try to incorporate staging variables into the definition of CFS (as already exists with HIV patients).

There is already international acceptance of the definition of CFS as laid down by the Centers for Disease Control (CDC) in the USA. To further refine the criteria by dividing the disease into stages or phases would help eliminate some of the variables and make immunological data more meaningful.

Hypothalamic and pituitary dysfunction

Some of the symptoms of CFS point to the involvement of the pituitary gland and the hypothalamic part of the brain. The neuropsychological symptoms include loss of concentrating ability, short-term memory loss, headaches and sleep disturbance. Control group studies have suggested that impaired cognitive function in CFS patients is a consequence of their condition.

Hypothalamic function and the level of serum prolactin have also been studied. It has been shown that CFS patients are markedly more sensitive to the effects of the chemical serotonin, which stimulates the production of prolactin.

Similarly, the angiotensin-vasopressin levels in CFS patients are disturbed. This affects the way the body handles water load and can account for the excessive thirst noted as a minor symptom in some CFS patients.

The brain controls the level of other chemicals in the

body. Corticotrophin and cortisol levels are disturbed in some CFS patients and this can mimic adrenal insufficiency, suggesting a possible central mechanism for both fatigue and immune dysfunction. It has been speculated that a persisting viral infection could account for the disturbed hormone and neurotransmitter production seen in hypothalamic dysfunction.

Disturbed brainstem circulation

Abnormal cerebral blood flow has been demonstrated in a majority of CFS patients studied using a kind of X-ray technique called single photon emission computed tomography (SPECT). The resulting SPECT scans have shown perfusion defects to several areas of the brain, especially the brainstem, and also altered metabolism of cells. Whether this is a primary phenomenon is not clear, but neurotransmitter regulation could be disturbed as a result.

Those patients followed up with serial SPECT scans have shown changes over time. In other words, the SPECT scan abnormalities do not represent permanent changes in the brain, but rather a dynamic process. Like the immune system abnormalities they may improve during the course of the illness, and resolve completely.

Many of the symptoms in CFS are linked to the central nervous system (CNS). Headaches, balance disturbance and temperature regulation abnormalities are frequently cited. *And the muscle weakness which is such a prominent symptom may also have a central rather than a peripheral origin.* It is the perception of muscle weakness that is complained of, rather than the muscle wasting seen in other disorders (e.g. poliomyelitis).

The phenomenon of neurally mediated hypotension may also be relevant here. As discussed earlier, the compromised circulation may not be so severe as to cause syncope (fainting) but may affect cerebral blood flow with resultant perfusion defects.

Brain stem compression

Recent research has focused attention on neurological conditions in which the brain stem or upper portion of the spinal cord is squeezed within the surrounding canal. This occurs in two situations:

- cervical stenosis, where the spinal cord appears normal but is too narrow for the spinal cord. A condition called syringomyelia may develop, in which a cyst grows in the spinal canal, resulting in even greater pressure on the cord.
- Chiari malformation, where part of the brain extends beyond the base of the skull and presses on the brain stem and spinal cord.

The symptoms of brain stem compression include many of those associated with brain stem ischaemia (discussed above). They include headache in the back of the head (occipital region) that may radiate to the eyes, neck and shoulders. Muscle weakness, imbalance, memory impairment, visual disturbances, gastrointestinal problems, paraesthesia and chronic fatigue are also common.

The role of spinal surgery to relieve the pressure may sound drastic but, in severe cases, may well be justified. A full neurological assessment, including MRI scans and X-rays, will soon distinguish those cases in which surgical intervention may be of benefit.

Increased levels of enzymes

Angiotensin converting enzyme (ACE) is an example of a substance found in increased levels in CFS patients. Interestingly, it is also elevated in the condition sarcoidosis, which shares some of the same symptoms (fatigue, arthralgia and neurological dysfunction). If neurotransmitter regulation is disturbed in one such condition it may also be implicated in another, with an overlap of symptoms.

It is easy to see why there is such confusion about CFS,

and why cerebral involvement has long been suspected. Neurological involvement seems certain.

The role of infectious agents

Any or all of the above scenarios (abnormal immune response, hypothalamic and pituitary dysfunction, disturbed brainstem circulation, and increased levels of certain enzymes) may be caused by a viral (or other) infection. In fact, viral infection, together with another risk or trigger factor, still appears to be the most likely cause of the changes that result in CFS.

A recent Australian study has even suggested that CFS patients are genetically prone to the illness. A series of fatty acid changes have been found in CFS patients, indicating possible underlying genetic conditions that predispose them to viral infection. The changes were likened to the scenario where the dormant herpes virus has been activated to produce a cold sore in someone whose metabolism has changed.

Some cases of CFS follow in the wake of an acute illness from well-proven infection. Glandular fever (infectious mononucleosis) is usually caused by the Epstein-Barr virus (EBV) and its course can be followed not only clinically but serologically in the laboratory. In a minority of cases the symptoms can persist for several years, with exercise-related fatigue the predominant complaint. Other specific infectious causes include Lyme disease (caused by the bacterium *Borrelia burgdorferi*), Ross River virus, and acute Q fever (caused by the bacterium *Coxiella burnettii*).

In most cases the exact organism remains unknown. Researchers believe the most likely contenders belong to one of several families of viruses:

- enteroviruses (including polio, Coxsackie and echoviruses)
- herpes viruses (including herpes zoster)
- retroviruses

- other viruses (including cytomegalovirus, Ross River and rubella)
- non-viral (including Q fever).

Viral cultures may confirm the presence of a virus, but are not always diagnostic. The viruses and their qualities are discussed in more detail below.

Enteroviruses

Enteroviruses make up the largest group implicated in CFS. They include the Coxsackie and echoviruses (about 30 of each type), the polio viruses and hepatitis A. They may cause a wide spectrum of illnesses ranging from upper respiratory infections and gastroenteritis to severe life-threatening infections like meningitis and encephalitis. These latter serious illnesses are seen when there is inflammation of the spinal cord or brain tissue. There may also be involvement of muscles or heart (myocarditis and pericarditis), and other specific organs may be affected including liver (hepatitis), pancreas and thyroid gland.

Of course not all such infections go on to persist as CFS. But the very wide range of initial presentations needs to be considered in any patient presenting with symptoms suggestive of CFS. Remember that the majority (75 per cent) of CFS patients have a history of an acute viral-type illness.

Scrupulous standards of cleanliness with food preparation, handling and storage are essential to prevent viral (and bacterial) infection. Failure to practise basic hygiene and contamination of water supplies will increase the risk of enteroviral infection. Seawater polluted by sewage can cause food poisoning on a large scale via infected seafood (oysters, scallops etc.).

Infants can be another source of infection. Babies can be carriers of enteroviruses without having any symptoms of infection themselves. Adults handling nappies are at risk of catching or passing on the virus unless they are especially careful to wash and dry their hands thoroughly.

In most developed countries enteroviruses tend to thrive in the warmer months. High standards of hygiene mean that these populations have little natural immunity, other than by exposure and antibody production to a specific virus. If slight mutations occur and a new strain emerges there is no natural immunity within a community.

Hospitals are another obvious source of enteroviral (or other) infection. With open wounds, dirty dressings and air conditioning blowing out recycled air, one is not automatically safe in a clinical setting. And hospital staff are not always so careful. It is a sorry state of affairs that basic aseptic measures are less stringent than they used to be. Doctors and nurses in busy wards do not always wash their hands with antiseptic between patients. Barrier nursing is much less common these days. And there is a disturbing trend in some hospitals for nursing staff to discard their clean fresh uniforms for the less 'threatening' look of daytime street clothing.

With the easy availability of antibiotics to treat secondary infections, we have seen an alarming rise in the incidence of antibiotic-resistant bacteria in recent years. This is a worldwide problem and it is only a matter of time before we face major outbreaks of infection for which there is no cure. It cannot be emphasised too strongly that medical staff (both doctors and nurses) must remain constantly aware of the need for aseptic practices.

Enteroviruses possess a core or genetic code of ribonucleic acid (RNA). This viral nucleic acid has the function of invading a host cell and using the host cell's genetic apparatus to reproduce itself. Unlike some other viruses, the enterovirus is a poor replicator. It certainly produces more viruses, but they are imperfect copies of the original virus. The multiplication process continues and, with each successive generation of viruses, they become more and more imperfect, resulting in 'mutant forms'.

A practical example of a mutant form is the common influenza virus. Over several years the flu virus gradually mutates. This continues until the body's immune system is unable to recognise and challenge a virus which it was previously able to tackle. It has changed so much that antibodies previously formed are now no longer effective. For this reason the familiar flu vaccines vary slightly from year to year to take into account the tendency of a virus to mutate.

Herpes viruses

This group contains a number of viruses that can cause cold sores (herpes simplex), genital herpes and chickenpox (herpes zoster). The herpes simplex is not thought to be involved, but others in the herpes group have been definitely proven to be linked in some cases of CFS.

The reactivation of a dormant herpes zoster can, in later life, cause the unpleasant condition of shingles. The patient will almost certainly have had chickenpox when younger (even if only a mild case clinically) and the virus will remain for life. When the immune system is weakened, one of the trigger factors may present, the virus is no longer kept in check and shingles results.

The Epstein-Barr virus (EBV), another member of the herpes group, is known to cause infectious mononucleosis or glandular fever. It can be spread by saliva (hence the term 'kissing disease') and affects predominantly teenagers or young adults. Patients usually present with a very sore throat (extremely inflamed on examination), markedly swollen glands (either locally or more widespread) and a fever. Headaches are common and the young patient is frequently fatigued.

Glandular fever usually lasts at least three or four weeks and often longer. It is highly contagious and carriers of the disease can pass it on without developing it themselves. The patient's clinical course usually coincides with a large number of atypical lymphocytes (a type of white blood cell) seen on a blood film examination. In addition, a specific serological test is positive, although it may take some days to turn positive. If symptoms persist and glandular fever is suspected, the serology should be repeated.

Like the herpes zoster virus in chickenpox, the Epstein-Barr virus usually remains in the body for life. It is suppressed by cells of the immune system and most patients will develop specific antibodies to EBV which bestow a full degree of immunity.

Another, newer member of the herpes group to be implicated in CFS is the human herpes virus type 6/HHV-6. This was isolated by Dr Robert Gallo, the scientist involved in AIDS research at the National Cancer Institute in the USA. Initially Gallo did not establish a conclusive link, but more recent findings have suggested a possible connection.

Professor Tony Komaroff and his research team studied the blood taken from some of the patients who were known to have become ill as a result of the outbreak around Lake Tahoe. Their white blood cells showed cellular damage similar to that seen in cells infected with the HHV-6. It is thought that, like EBV, most patients come into contact with HHV-6 at an early age, after which it remains dormant in the body. The stimulus of some trigger factor (concurrent infection, stress) is believed to cause some immune system dysfunction, leading to a reactivation of the HHV-6.

HHV-6 may be responsible for glandular fever in some patients. Although not so common a cause as EBV, it may be more prone to reactivation. The possibility of it then progressing to the overproduction of cytokines, with symptoms of CFS resulting, is a very real one indeed.

The nuclear code of a herpes virus is made of deoxyribonucleic acid (DNA). Its replication within a host cell is similar to that of the enteroviruses, except that they have RNA instead of DNA as their viral nucleic acid. The DNA present in the herpes group has important practical implications.

A major development has been the introduction in recent years of anti-viral drugs. These are only effective, however, against some of the DNA-containing herpes viruses. A drug that is effective against the DNA-containing viruses will not work on an RNA-containing virus, meaning that there is no drug treatment for the (RNA-containing) enteroviruses at present.

The main anti-viral drug, acyclovir, is particularly useful in severe cases of herpes zoster. This may be a case of chickenpox that has developed the complication of life-threatening pneumonia. Or it may be a case of shingles in an older patient where the nerve involved could result in the loss of vision in one eye.

Acyclovir is active only against the DNA replication within the cell. It has no detrimental effect on the healthy host cell. Instead, its action is highly specific and it only works when the virus is actively multiplying.

There is at present no indication to use acyclovir in cases of CFS, even where Epstein-Barr virus is thought to be involved. Even if more anti-viral drugs are developed (for use against RNA-containing viruses), their use in the treatment of CFS remains uncertain. The implication, yet again, is that it is the over-active immune response, rather than the virus itself, that causes the symptoms.

Retroviruses

Retroviruses are characterised by the presence of an enzyme called 'reverse transcriptase'. This unique enzyme is involved in the replication of the virus once it has invaded a normal cell.

The most sinister quality of retroviruses is their ability to attack the T4 helper lymphocyte cells—an integral part of one's immune system. Two types of the human T-cell leukaemia virus (HTLV1 and HTLV2) have been implicated in leukaemia and other neurological diseases. And the most studied virus of our time, the human immunodeficiency virus (HIV), has been established as the cause of acquired immune deficiency syndrome (AIDS).

The enormous global significance of the AIDS outbreak of the 1980s and 1990s has led to great advances in anti-retroviral therapy. There are three differing mechanisms of actions for these drugs. The most commonly used is the nucleoside analogue sub-group. These drugs all inhibit the same viral enzyme 'reverse transcriptase' and include zidovudine, didanosone and zalcitabine. Other sub-groups include the non-nucleoside reverse transcriptase inhibitors (e.g. nevirapine) and the protease inhibitors (e.g. ritonavir).

Anti-retroviral therapy is associated with increased survival and improved quality of life in patients with symptomatic HIV infection. Used either as monotherapy or, increasingly, in combination, they have been shown to reduce the progression to full-blown AIDS.

Evidence that viral replication occurs continuously throughout the asymptomatic period provides a rationale for early therapy in HIV infection. But problems of viral resistance to one drug are common and combination therapy from the start is becoming the preferred treatment.

Anti-retroviral therapy is associated with some major side-effects, especially in more advanced HIV infection. Peripheral neuropathy and haematological abnormalities (anaemia and neutropenia) are two such problems. And the interactions between the anti-retrovirals and the many other drugs given prophylactically in HIV infection mean that patients need careful monitoring, including frequent measurements of their T4 helper cell levels.

There is no real likelihood of anti-retroviral drugs being of use in CFS. Even if a retrovirus were isolated, the same reasons for not using acyclovir in a chronic Epstein-Barr viral infection would apply. The body's exaggerated immune response appears to be the main problem in CFS. Any benefit from an anti-viral (or anti-retroviral) drug would, I suspect, depend on it being used in the early stages of the infection; that is, before the symptoms or sequelae of CFS became clinically obvious.

Other viruses

Australian studies have shown that CFS can follow from Ross River virus (RRV) infection. But, interestingly, RRV does not appear to be neurotropic; that is, the virus is not known to affect brain tissue. Yet many researchers believe that CFS has its effect within the brain. And other viruses that are linked to CFS, like EBV, are known to be able to infect brain tissue. Certainly the evidence is that there is no long-term damage to the brain tissue. But at present we await further results of trials that compare patients with RRV to other control CFS patients who have a history of acute, recent-onset glandular fever or Q fever (see below).

Both cytomegalovirus (CMV) and rubella have also been associated with the development of CFS. But their involvement would appear to be as just one trigger factor. Once more the evidence would suggest it is the immune response they cause rather than anything specifically to do with the virus itself.

Non-viral infection

Viruses are not the only types of infectious agents to trigger an abnormal immune response. Professor Barrie Marmion, a microbiologist in Adelaide, has shown that patients with acute Q fever, which is caused by a small intracellular bacterium (*Coxiella burnettii*) could, in 15–20 per cent of cases, go on to develop a fatigue syndrome similar to CFS (termed QFS).

Q fever is an important occupational hazard for workers in the meat and livestock industry, with about 1000 cases reported in Australia each year. The organism is spread in dust after the slaughter of an infected animal. Symptoms of

QFS include inappropriate incapacitating fatigue, myalgia, nausea, headache and night sweats. There may also be disturbed sleeping patterns together with changes in mood and mental concentration. A small proportion can go on to develop chronic hepatitis, endocarditis or osteitis (bone infection).

Symptoms are either continuous from the acute attack or occur as a relapse up to a year after the acute attack. QFS lasts at least two years but more usually persists for five to six years. The chance of developing the Q fatigue syndrome is much less if the acute Q fever is treated immediately with doxycycline (an antibiotic to which the causative organism is sensitive).

Doxycycline is a commonly prescribed antibiotic, generally well tolerated with few side-effects. It is used with safety in patients with chronic bronchitis or severe acne, but it must not be given to children.

Abnormal staphylococci

Recent research (1998) at the University of Newcastle (Australia) has revealed that the normal bacterial flora may be replaced by certain abnormal microorganisms in CFS patients. Professor Tim Roberts, Dr Hugh Dunstan and Dr Henry Butt have shown that atypical staphylococcal bacteria produce toxins that can damage cell walls and affect normal cellular function and absorptive processes. This supports earlier work at the University of Goteborg (Sweden) where Professor Carl Gottfries has produced a vaccine to counteract staphylococcal infection.

The Swedish and Australian studies give hope that a future clinical treatment may be based on the use of such a vaccine. Already, in experimental trials, Professor Gottfries has shown the beneficial results from using a vaccine to counteract the effect of staphylococcal toxins in a group of patients who have suffered CFS for ten or more years. In more than half those vaccinated over a four to six year period there has been demonstrable improvement in their clinical symptoms.

Summary

It is my belief that no one particular virus is implicated in CFS. A more likely scenario is that the temporary immune suppression resulting from one viral infection may allow another infection to take hold. The resultant stimulus to the immune system causes damage or hyperactivity in one's immune response. It is like an electrical circuit being overloaded. The immune system either cannot cope or it overreacts in some way that requires an enormous amount of ongoing energy at the cellular level.

There is also the possibility that one virus may reactivate a dormant virus that has been present for years—somewhat similar to the chickenpox virus (herpes varicella) lying dormant for years and being reactivated later in life to cause shingles. A temporarily abnormal immune system, perhaps made more susceptible by physical or mental stress, will allow the chain of events to occur that results in the virus being resurrected in another form—perhaps a form that throws our immune responses into 'overdrive' and produces the symptoms of CFS.

Lastly, the role of endotoxins in producing the symptoms of CFS must be considered. The ongoing research in Australia and Sweden implicates the presence of abnormal staphylococci as part of an atypical flora in CFS patients. The resultant toxins may well disrupt normal cellular function, with the production of cytokines leading to the clinical features of CFS.

Symptoms of CFS

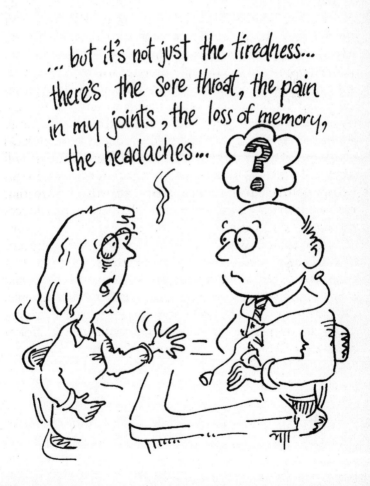

... but it's not just the tiredness... there's the sore throat, the pain in my joints, the loss of memory, the headaches...

Although CFS has been recognised and written about for many years there is still a need to define what it actually means.

'Chronic fatigue syndrome' is an unfortunate label. It tends to trivialise what is a quite devastating illness. Until there is more known about the underlying pathophysiology there is no point in changing the name. Undoubtedly research will eventually throw more light on its aetiology. However, to change the name without scientific justification will cause confusion and undermine the progress that has already been made.

The International CFS Study Group—consisting of researchers from the USA, Australia, the United Kingdom, Canada, Italy, Sweden, and the Netherlands—met in September 1993. The meeting was convened by the Centers for Disease Control and Prevention (CDC) in the USA to review the definition of 'chronic fatigue syndrome'. A conceptual framework and guidelines were established by which the illness could be diagnosed and the collection of data standardised so as to give a greater understanding of the illness.

From that meeting it was agreed that CFS is a subset of the population with prolonged fatigue. 'Prolonged fatigue' was defined as 'self-reported persistent fatigue lasting one month or longer' while 'chronic fatigue' (of which CFS is also a subset) was defined as 'self-reported persistent or relapsing fatigue lasting six or more consecutive months'.

Since fatigue is associated with a variety of other medical and psychiatric conditions it was necessary to clarify and update the definition of chronic fatigue syndrome.

A case of chronic fatigue syndrome is defined by the presence of the following:

i *clinically evaluated, unexplained, persistent or relapsing chronic fatigue that is of new or definite onset (has not been lifelong); is not the result of ongoing exertion; is not substantially alleviated by rest; and results in a substantial reduction in previous levels of occupational, social or personal activities; and*

ii *the concurrent occurrence of four or more of the following symptoms, all of which must have persisted or recurred during six or more consecutive months of illness and must not have predated the fatigue: self-reported impairment in short-term memory or concentration severe enough to cause substantial reduction in previous levels of occupational, educational, social or personal activities; sore throat with tender cervical or axillary lymph nodes; muscle pain; multi-joint pain without swelling or redness; headache of a new type, pattern or severity; unrefreshing sleep; and post-exertional malaise lasting more than 24 hours.*

The Study Group offered two major classification categories: chronic fatigue syndrome (as defined above) and idiopathic chronic fatigue. Idiopathic chronic fatigue is defined as 'clinically evaluated unexplained chronic fatigue that fails to meet the criteria for chronic fatigue syndrome'.

With a condition like CFS, it is important that any definitions or laid down criteria are not seen as inflexible. While it is crucial to have guidelines one must be aware that the range of symptoms in CFS is diverse. No two patients with CFS will have the same set of symptoms, although there will of course be overlap with the main features of profound fatigue, muscle aching and brain-related features present in all cases.

For ease of discussion, I have divided the symptoms of CFS into three main sections:
- Muscle fatigue
- Brain malfunction
- Secondary symptoms (present, to a greater or lesser degree).

Muscle fatigue

The most characteristic and profound symptom, found in 100 per cent of CFS patients, is muscle fatigue induced by minimal exertion. The exertion needed to produce fatigue may be so minimal that even the slightest task becomes a major challenge. Many patients find that merely getting up in the morning, showering and dressing deplete their limited energy stores. They may need to lie down after breakfast in order to recoup enough strength to proceed cautiously with their day's duties, curtailed as they may be. When CFS is at its worst the fatigue is present without even trying to move about. It is this severity of fatigue that leaves a patient bed-bound and reliant on symptomatic relief.

The most accurate way of describing muscle involvement is to think of it on three levels. At rest, there may be no obvious discomfort. On exercising or simply moving about, you will notice the muscles becoming fatigued. If the exertion is stopped and you rest, then the muscle fatigue will often decrease without severe after-effects. But if you continue the exertion there will come a point at which the fatigue turns into discomfort or the muscle becomes quite painful.

In the early stages of CFS the most distressing aspect is being unable to predict how far you can go (literally!). Provided you stop and rest at the first feelings of fatigue, then relief will occur and the symptoms subside, often without any medication. But if you push yourself beyond the fatigue warning level, then the symptoms will persist, only responding to enforced (and sometimes prolonged) rest and anti-inflammatory medication. The more you have over-exerted yourself the longer it will take for the muscles to return to normal.

A fairly common scenario is when the patient is out shopping, gardening or socialising. It is very tempting to ignore what, to the normal person, would seem like minimal symptoms of fatigue, similar to those we all experience at the end of a long day. But where the healthy person is relieved at getting home, changing into casual clothes and slippers and putting the feet up, the CFS patient more frequently heads for bed and hopes the muscular discomfort will resolve and not affect the following day's activities.

Another frustrating element of muscle fatigue is the often 'delayed relapse'. This may occur up to 24 hours after exertion, so it is difficult to know how much one can do (e.g. walking) if the effect is not immediate. My own experience has been that, with improvement, the immediate fatigue has become less difficult to cope with. Instead, I have paid the price with symptoms occurring a day later and have had to plan my activities accordingly.

If there is a risk of doing too much one day, you simply have to be ruthless in refusing an invitation or setting a limit on your activities. Even if you accomplish more than you expected without any immediate ill-effect, there is a strong possibility that you may spend the entire next day in bed, after a delayed response. But it takes time to predict one's capabilities and to acknowledge one's limitations. I am still learning!

It is the severe limitations that make CFS so debilitating. Simple tasks like a short walk (e.g. to the letterbox) may bring on the fatigue, and repetitive tasks over a longer period (e.g. gardening or sport) become simply impossible. The fact that we are used to doing all these relatively mundane things makes no difference. If the warning signs are ignored, then there will be a prolonged period of immobility to restore the energy levels and try to learn from our mistakes.

The early symptoms of muscle fatigue are similar to those seen in a patient who is convalescing after a viral infection. Post-viral malaise or fatigue is a common feature of glandular fever, for example; patients find they need more rest in the weeks or months following infection. A prolonged recovery is often a feature of glandular fever and reintroduction of normal activities must be very gradual to avoid a relapse.

The greatest problem with CFS is that this situation persists for so long. Even if you learn to obey the warning symptoms there are always the situations where, because you feel so much better, there is the temptation to try just a little harder. In a normal situation this would not create a problem, but in CFS sufferers it may result in a period of extended bed rest and enforced immobility.

Not surprisingly, most patients become depressed by the very severe limitations imposed by CFS. Some days it will happen that, no sooner than having bathed, shaved and dressed oneself to start the day, the fatigue will be so bad that it will be necessary to lie down for another hour or so to try to recoup some energy. As the illness progresses, the patient comes to sense whether it will be a good or a bad day by how he or she feels after breakfast. The mornings are usually the worst part of the day, but some days are worse than others.

Despite the periods of prolonged immobility there is seldom any muscle wasting. This is an important feature of CFS, which distinguishes it from other conditions such as myopathies and poliomyelitis. However, extended periods of bed rest should be avoided if possible and a gentle program of mobilisation incorporated into the daily routine.

All muscles can be affected. The muscles of the upper and lower limbs are probably the most frequently involved, but muscles of the neck and chest are also susceptible. Even tendons are sometimes sore depending on the activity that has occurred. And the small muscles of the eye can make reading for any length of time another cause of muscle fatigue (and possible headaches).

Fasciculations (or muscle twitchings) are also more common in CFS patients. This may involve any muscle group but it is more likely to be seen in muscles of the upper and lower limbs, especially the biceps and the muscles of the hand. And the small muscles that control the eyelids may be prone to involuntary flickering (or blepharospasm), which is a sign of fatigue and can be aggravated by bright light.

It is important to remember it may well be our perception of muscle weakness and pain that is altered in CFS. This could account for the exaggerated response of our bodies to what would normally be a trivial amount of exercise or activity. The role of ischaemia or compression of the brain stem has already been discussed (under 'Aetiology').

Treatment of muscle fatigue

- *Rest* is the most obvious remedy for exercise-induced muscle fatigue. This may not always mean bed rest and will be a matter of trial and error. Simply lying with the feet elevated will bring relief in cases of fatigue where pain has not yet become a feature.
- *Hydrotherapy* is ideal, provided the muscles are not painful. I have found that a hot bath on getting up in the morning will help to mobilise the muscles, further aided by a herbal or mineral bath gel (such as Dencorub or Badedas). Gently flex and extend all joints, also rotating them if possible. Follow this with stretching exercises of both upper and lower limbs, concluding with stretches of shoulder girdles and lower back. Then rest, allowing the warmth to penetrate the muscles for a further five to ten minutes.
- A *non-steroidal anti-inflammatory drug* may be necessary if the muscle fatigue does not respond to the above measures, or if the muscles are feeling painful. These must always be taken *after meals* and should be used only with the approval of your general practitioner. These drugs are all capable of causing gastric irritation and possibly bleeding, blood disorders, nausea and rashes. Some are available as an ointment or spray—an obvious advantage if there is a contra-indication to taking them orally.
- An *analgesic* is an alternate, or additional, medication. Drugs such as paracetamol, with or without codeine, are ideal in milder cases where an anti-inflammatory is not required or is unavailable. But it is important not to

exceed the recommended maximum dosage, as both these constituents have side-effects. In severe pain, an analgesic (but not aspirin) can be used in addition to an anti-inflammatory drug.

Paracetamol in large dosage over a prolonged period can cause damage to both the kidneys and the liver. Codeine will cause constipation in many patients, even at moderate dosage. Other side-effects of codeine include nausea, drowsiness and light-headedness.

Aspirin is an extremely valuable drug in CFS. It is an excellent analgesic and, unlike paracetamol, has some anti-inflammatory action. It should therefore not be taken with any other anti-inflammatory drug, but can be combined with codeine for maximal analgesic effect.

Like other anti-inflammatory drugs, aspirin should not be taken if there is a history of gastric irritation, bleeding or ulcer. And it must not be given to children under the age of thirteen.

- Other drugs include *tricyclic antidepressants*. These have been shown to be of benefit in many chronic musculoskeletal and neurological conditions. As they may cause sedation they are best given at night, combined with an analgesic or non-steroidal anti-inflammatory drug for maximal effect. Depression is frequently a secondary problem in CFS, so the benefits of such a preparation may be twofold.

- *Alternative therapies* for muscle fatigue include acupuncture, physiotherapy, anti-oxidant therapy, herbal medicine, homeopathy, and transcendental medication. These will be discussed in further detail in Chapter 5.

Brain malfunction

Before I elaborate on this particular aspect of CFS I should stress that the so-called 'malfunction' of the brain is totally reversible in the vast majority of patients. Some of the most troublesome symptoms of CFS are due to cerebral involvement, but they are fortunately among the first to subside.

As discussed in the previous chapter, various changes have been noted in the brains of CFS patients. Specifically hypothalamic and pituitary dysfunction have been reported, with the implication of disturbed hormone and neurotransmitter production. Disturbed blood flow to the brainstem has also been demonstrated, resulting in perfusion defects.

Despite there being obvious brain malfunction, none of these effects has been shown to cause permanent damage to brain tissue. There has been no evidence of any dementing process and the features of intellectual malfunction have fluctuated in severity. The symptoms of cerebral involvement have usually corresponded to the relapses seen after episodes of increased physical and mental activity.

Although the term 'myalgic encephalomyelitis' (ME) has often been used as an alternative name to CFS, there has never been any firm evidence that encephalitis (or inflammation of the brain tissues) is actually taking place. That is one very good reason why 'chronic fatigue syndrome'—although trivialising the illness—is a better term at this stage than 'myalgic encephalomyelitis'.

It is well known that some of the common viruses are capable of crossing the blood-brain barrier and replicating inside brain cells. Measles, mumps, rubella, chickenpox and Epstein-Barr are all able to affect the production of cytokines and neurotransmitters.

All these viruses, and the enteroviruses as well, are therefore able to increase or decrease the level of neurotransmitters. These are basically chemicals that transmit messages within the nervous system and so control sleep requirements, mood changes and energy levels. It is for this reason that many scientists believe the 'fatigue' part of CFS emanates from the brain and not the muscles. The 'perception' of fatigue may well be more relevant than the actual muscles themselves, which are quite normal.

The effects of viruses stimulating the production of neuro-transmitters and other immune chemicals are of great importance. The neurotransmitter called serotonin is made from the amino acid tryptophan. Increased levels of sero-tonin in the brain can occur from its uptake into the nerve endings being blocked by certain drugs or possibly the effects of certain viruses. Imbalanced levels of serotonin are known to be relevant in disturbances of mood, sleep patterns, memory, appetite and sexual behaviour.

There are other immune chemical imbalances that may result from persisting viral stimulation. In particular, increased amounts of the chemical interferon may have a direct effect on mental functioning; and there is no reason why mitochondrial ('power-houses' within individual cells) dysfunction due to viral influences should be less important in brain tissue than it is in muscle.

In short, there are many chemical changes occurring at cell level in the brains of CFS patients. But the actual structure of the brain tissue is not affected. There is nothing of a degenerative or destructive nature taking place. The brain cells are normal but are made to malfunction because it is the chemical make-up of the fluids surrounding them that is temporarily affected in CFS.

Common symptoms of brain malfunction and their treatment

Impairment of short-term memory

This symptom occurs in about 80 per cent of patients and it is one of the most frustrating symptoms of all, especially if you have always been fortunate enough to have a memory like an elephant. It becomes apparent on trying to recall names, especially of people you've not known for a long time. It can be annoying socially, but explaining the situation frankly is usually the best policy. Long-term memory is (thankfully) unaffected. This situation occurs in all of us with age, and it occurs prematurely in patients with Alzheimer's disease. The difference in CFS is that the situation does improve with time.

Memory for facts and figures is likewise affected only if recent events are involved. Its duration corresponds with the amount of time the patient has been suffering from CFS. Fortunately, you can usually look things up and recommit them to memory. As the illness improves, this short-term memory is one of the first things to return. But needless to say, it is imperative to keep an updated diary and make plenty of notes.

Impaired concentration is an allied symptom, not always present to the same degree. However, any prolonged period of mental activity (reading, writing, attending lectures) can produce quite profound fatigue in some patients. The symptom appears to be at its worst in the early stages of the illness and, like short-term memory, tends to improve with each remission.

Headaches

Headaches occur to a significant degree in about 75 per cent of patients. But headaches are a common symptom of many illnesses so it is important to exclude other causes before blaming CFS. Migraines, high blood pressure and sinusitis are some of the other common causes of headaches, which can be easily diagnosed by talking to one's GP.

Of those CFS patients who suffer headaches, about a third complain that they are frequent and severe. They may be bilateral or unilateral, throbbing or dull, and tend to respond poorly to common analgesics. In a large number of sufferers they are migrainous in nature and should be treated accordingly.

Resting in a quiet, darkened room, taking a stronger type of analgesic (containing codeine) and keeping up your fluid input usually helps. In less severe cases some patients have had relief from evening primrose oil, while the more severe headaches should be treated along the lines of a conventional migraine attack. Some of the newer specific drugs like sumatriptan, which act on the serotonin receptors in the brain, may be required in extreme cases.

Avoidance of known aggravating factors in the diet is also important. In particular, cheese, red wine and chocolate should be reduced or eliminated if headaches are known to follow their ingestion.

Other headaches reported by CFS patients are more likely to be related to muscular strain. The neck muscles can produce headaches as can the small muscles of the eye. Prolonged reading or bookwork can often precipitate both general fatigue and headache due to over-use of the eye muscles.

Another frequent cause of headache, in both CFS patients and the general population, is referred pain from the cervical spine. A history of injury (sporting, whiplash) may be obtained and a clinical examination will soon reveal which nerves are involved. An X-ray may well show some cervical disc degeneration that may have been present for years, yet it only causes nerve root irritation (and referred pain) intermittently.

Anti-inflammatory drugs are of great help in this situation. In severe cases a cervical collar may be of help, but the condition does not usually require this rather conspicuous form of treatment. Physiotherapy and acupuncture can also be of benefit. Injecting the nerve root is another temporary form of treatment, while surgery to remove or decompress the offending disc is another option in cases of persistent chronic pain.

Correct diagnosis of the cause of a headache is essential. If a specific reason can be found, it can usually be treated quite independently of any other symptoms of CFS. And remember, having CFS does not mean you cannot develop headaches from some other totally unrelated cause.

Autonomic-related symptoms

The autonomic nervous system is especially affected by CFS and this leads to a wide range of symptoms, which at first may seem unrelated. About 70 per cent of all CFS patients report one or more symptoms that fall into this category. Unlike the nerves that supply and direct muscle and joint movement, we have little control over the autonomic nervous system, which consists of two complementary systems known as the 'sympathetic' and the 'parasympathetic' pathways. These have opposing actions, are controlled by centres in the brainstem and act to maintain the body in a state of 'equilibrium'. The nervous pathways supply the heart and blood vessels, and are involved in the control of bowel and bladder function as well as helping to regulate body temperature.

i *Heart and blood vessels:* An increase in sympathetic nervous activity leads to an increase in pulse rate (tachycardia) and the sensation of the heart beating more strongly (palpitations). Blood pressure can be affected in a number of ways. It may become elevated, or, because of the dilation of the larger blood vessels, there may be a postural hypotensive effect, where the blood pressure actually falls when the patient changes from lying or sitting to a standing position. The blood flow to the brain is compromised (due to the 'pooling' effect of gravity) and the patient feels faint or light-headed as a result.

Certain drugs can help to neutralise the effects of an overactive sympathetic nervous system. In particular, the b-blocking group are very helpful in controlling tachycardia and palpitations. However, they must only be taken as prescribed and only after any other cardiac problems have been excluded by your doctor. But the side-effects of b-blockers can be a problem; especially in higher dosage when they can aggravate the symptoms of CFS and also drop the blood pressure, which is one of their main therapeutic uses.

It is equally important to avoid substances that cause palpitations and tachycardia. Caffeine (mostly in coffee) and the drug 'pseudoephedrine' (found in many decongestant preparations) are two common offenders, so should be used with care. Excess caffeine late in the day will frequently cause sleep disturbances which, in themselves, are another problem (see below).

ii *Temperature regulation:* Your natural body 'thermostat' is the hypothalamus part of the brain. Apart from its effect on autonomic control, the hypothalamus has also been implicated by its tendency to suffer from reduced blood flow in CFS patients.

In fact, CFS patients have reported an increased awareness of body temperature that is unassociated with measurable abnormalities in thyroid function or core body temperature. Many patients complain of being especially sensitive to extremes of temperature, a finding also noted in multiple sclerosis. The natural tendency to sweat (to reduce body temperature) can be exacerbated in CFS patients, especially after they have overexerted themselves physically or mentally.

I have found that my fatigue is aggravated by a hot or humid climate. The last few summers have been spent largely indoors in an air-conditioned environment. I would recommend that CFS sufferers put temperature control of their homes as a high priority.

The effect of the autonomic nervous system on the more peripheral blood vessels may be to cause a reduced blood supply to the skin. This can lead to the obvious problems of cold hands and feet, as well as producing a marked facial pallor. Some of these peripheral symptoms may be exacerbated by b-blocking drugs. Cold weather and inhaling cigarette smoke are other aggravating factors that can worsen the symptoms.

Keeping warm in winter is obviously important. Sensible layered clothing is ideal, and it is best to keep the temperature of your home comfortably warm (but not hot). It is advisable to stimulate the circulation and maintain muscle tone by walking at least several times a week. If you cannot walk, due to a relapse, then passive exercises in bed are useful. If walking outdoors, thick woollen socks, comfortable walking boots, a scarf and a jacket will all help to retain body warmth. The benefits of a walking routine are invaluable, providing you have learnt how far you can exert yourself without producing profound fatigue as an after-effect.

During the winter months it is sensible to warm the bed with an electric blanket or a hot water bottle. The use of a duvet (continental quilt) or 'doona' is recommended because it is light yet warm. It is easier to flex and extend the joints and to maintain muscle tone with lighter bed-clothing. But the quilt must not be equivalent to more than two blankets or overheating can occur. Blankets may be better for some people in that there is often better distribution of heat. It is certainly easier to control bed warmth as you can throw off a blanket but cannot readily adjust a doona.

iii *Irritable bowel syndrome:* This troublesome set of symptoms includes stomach pain, nausea, alteration in bowel habit and bloatedness. It is a fairly common syndrome among the general population with an incidence of about 15 per cent. But the incidence among CFS sufferers is twice that.

The aetiology is uncertain, with probably a number of contributing factors. We know it can be triggered by an attack of gastroenteritis in some patients, while it is a stress-related complaint in others. In yet another group, food intolerance or allergy has been implicated. In all these patients there is the common link of the autonomic nerve supply to the gastrointestinal tract.

The muscles of the bowel wall are supplied by nerves of the autonomic system. An imbalance between sympathetic and parasympathetic pathways could well lead to rhythmic incoordination; the resulting disorderly muscle propulsions would certainly account for many of the symptoms of 'irritable bowel syndrome'.

Two other parts of the gastrointestinal tract can be affected by muscular spasms or incoordination. This can occur quite independently of the irritable bowel syndrome, and both conditions are more common in CFS sufferers than in the general population. They may well be more localised variants of the irritable bowel syndrome, without the multitude of symptoms that name implies:

Proctalgia fugax is an extremely painful cramp-like sensation in the anal muscle. It tends to affect young adults, usually male, and can last for between five minutes and half an hour, before gradually subsiding. It is infrequent, usually nocturnal, and can be relieved somewhat by dilating the anus or having a normal bowel motion. A warm bath may also help and a painkiller can be used if the symptoms persist.

Oesophageal spasms have also been reported. These cause difficulty with swallowing (dysphagia) and are usually self-limiting. However, they will need investigation should they become frequent. The opinion of a gastro-enterologist should be sought and an oesophagoscopy may well be advised.

As there are so many facets to irritable bowel syndrome it will be dealt with in more detail under Secondary Problems later in the chapter. But it is important to emphasise that changes in bowel habits in association with any bleeding from the rectum is certainly *not* irritable bowel syndrome and may be indicative of a more serious condition. Cancer of the bowel may mimic some of the symptoms of irritable bowel, and therefore you must not assume that it is the latter problem.

Indeed, I should stress that many of the individual symptoms of CFS could in fact be due to more sinister conditions. Even if CFS has been diagnosed, it is imperative that the patient is aware of any new or unusual symptoms, and that they be reported to the doctor so that a thorough examination and screening can be carried out.

iv *Bladder dysfunction:* As with the bowel, the muscles of the bladder wall are supplied by nerves of the autonomic system. The bladder's emptying mechanism is specifically involved and any incoordination can lead to the clinical picture of an 'irritable bladder'.

Fortunately only a minority of CFS patients are so affected. However, with age, muscle tone weakens and poor bladder control can result. Frequency of micturition (bladder emptying), getting up at night to pass urine, and the sensation of incomplete emptying of the bladder are all seen in CFS patients of both sexes.

A complicating factor in men is the prostate gland. Inflammation or enlargement may cause problems with passing urine. An enlarged prostate is found in most older men. Obviously the gland must be clinically assessed, with urine and blood tests and possibly X-rays, to be sure that the gland is not causing symptoms in its own right.

In women the problems of pelvic floor laxity can lead to urinary incontinence. Sudden coughing or increasing of intra-abdominal pressure can cause a 'bladder leak' due to incompetence of the bladder sphincter mechanism. This is seen especially in post-menopausal women where the lack of oestrogen causes the shrinking or atrophy of the tissues surrounding the vagina and the urethra. But, as in men with bladder problems, the urine must be examined for infection and the whole urinary tract may need to be examined radiologically with an IVP (intravenous pyelogram) or visualised by a urologist by means of a cystoscopy, where a small fibre optic instrument is inserted into the bladder via the urethra.

Assuming the absence of prostatic, renal and bladder pathology, both men and women can benefit greatly from pelvic floor exercises. These can be practised by stopping micturition mid-stream and starting again. By doing this several times while emptying the bladder, and repeating the exercise at regular intervals, the resultant muscle sphincter tone is increased and the bladder control improved.

v *Micturition syncope:* In point (i) ('Heart and blood vessels'), I discussed the drop in blood pressure that can occur on changing position, leading to the patient feeling faint. This effect, combined with the autonomic nerve involvement in bladder emptying, can cause the alarming symptom of micturition syncope. Typically this affects middle-aged to elderly males. The patient gets up in the middle of the night to pass urine and, while emptying the bladder, feels light-headed and faints on the bathroom floor.

Micturition syncope is by no means common in CFS patients. However, it appears to occur more frequently in this group than in the general population. Getting up slowly from the lying position helps to minimise the risk, as does sitting on the toilet if there is any feeling of faintness.

Balance disturbance

Balance disturbance is another frequent symptom of brain involvement and occurs in about 75 per cent of CFS patients. Some are affected greatly indeed. Rather than a true case of 'vertigo', where the patient reports a sensation of the external world revolving around him or her or of revolving around space, it is more a case of disturbed equilibrium.

My own situation involved a feeling of unsteadiness on walking down a flight of stairs. It was almost like having had too much to drink. I was forced to cling to a rail or banister for help. Oddly there was never a problem going up the stairs, only when coming down. This was a fairly early symptom that still persists to this day, although it is thankfully less severe.

Other patients have noted similar symptoms, with minor variations. For example, some have reported a feeling of imbalance on getting up suddenly, but this could well be allied to a drop in blood pressure due to a change in position. We know the inner ear structures and the cerebellum are involved in maintaining normal body equilibrium, so a temporary lack of blood supply (ischaemia) could well be involved.

Patients who have complained of severe, persisting

balance disturbance are a significant sub-group. They have often relayed a story of a viral inner ear infection (labyrinthitis) that has been a trigger factor in the development of their CFS. They obviously have special needs and are at much greater risk of falling. The infective link in this situation is of special interest.

As with other symptoms, the cause of disturbed balance should be carefully examined. Only a thorough neurological examination, with possible referral to an ear, nose and throat specialist, will exclude other more sinister causes. This is a symptom that is common to a good many conditions and some of them (e.g. an early brain tumour) require accurate diagnosis and appropriate treatment.

Sleep disturbances

About two-thirds of all CFS patients report changes in their sleeping patterns. Almost all patients require increased sleep, especially early in the course of the illness. Even those who have thrived on five or six hours' sleep at night for many years may find they require twice that amount of sleep or even more before they can function during the day.

One of the most frequent complaints from CFS patients is that they wake feeling unrefreshed, no matter how many hours they may have slept. The vast majority of patients find the mornings are their most difficult period and that simply getting up and about can produce the most profound fatigue on 'bad' days. The increased demand for sleep may also reflect the quality of sleep itself.

We know that sleep is divided into two main types. The 'dream'-type sleep associated with rapid eye movements is known as REM sleep and is the more superficial type, while the non-REM sleep or 'orthodox' type is deep sleep which occurs for longer phases. We regularly alternate between the two types of sleep throughout the night, with dream sleep occupying about a quarter of the total time we are asleep. The first few hours of sleep are generally the most important.

It is imperative that CFS patients accept the fact that their bodies require more sleep. This is one of the features of CFS that patients cannot fight against. It is apparent that the enormous dissipation of energy that occurs at all levels means their systems need time to recover and replenish those energy stores.

I mentioned earlier that both the brainstem and the hypothalamus are the sleep-controlling centres of the brain. These regions are thought to be involved in the aetiology of CFS. They are affected by both impaired perfusion (blood flow) and the circulation of certain cytokines triggered by the immune system overreacting to an infectious agent. It is no surprise then that the CFS patient has an increased need for sleep and, frequently, a coexistent abnormality in sleep patterns. These include:

i *Difficulty in falling asleep:* This is often anxiety-related and affects a major proportion of the population. But it is a common symptom in CFS patients and probably relates to many of the uncertainties of this condition.

There are many helpful ways to induce sleep. We shall look at these in more detail in Chapter 6. Creating the right environment, relaxation techniques and the avoidance of caffeine and other stimulants are all important.

If the problem persists, then the judicious use of a mild hypnotic (sleeping pill) will often re-establish a satisfactory sleeping pattern. The most commonly prescribed group are the short- or intermediate-acting benzodiazepines. But these must be used only as instructed and they are not intended for long-term use.

ii *Waking frequently during the night:* Physical symptoms can account for this and it is not, of course, restricted to CFS patients. For example, patients with arthritic conditions are frequently affected due to painful joints. In CFS patients, night-time symptoms frequently include muscular aches or pains and headaches. Less common causes of sleeplessness include bladder irritability, proctalgia fugax and night sweats.

The individual problems should be treated symptomatically. For example, an anti-inflammatory drug and/or a codeine containing analgesic is the best way to stop muscular pain. Local heat and gentle massage may be sufficient in milder cases where the ache has not turned to pain.

It is wise to avoid caffeine for six hours before bedtime and also to restrict fluid intake late at night. This will reduce the possibility of bladder problems. And a warm herbal bath is helpful for both muscular symptoms and to prevent proctalgia fugax.

Night sweats are distressing and a sign that your temperature-regulating mechanism is disturbed. Bed-clothing should be light and easily adjustable. Blankets may be preferable to a doona if the latter makes the bed too warm. Central heating must be switched off at night for at least seven or eight hours. There should be fresh air circulating via an open window. It is the bed that should be warm rather than the whole room.

When there is chronic pain or discomfort your doctor may also consider the use of an antidepressant drug at night. Usually one of the tricyclic group works best and can be used in association with an anti-inflammatory or analgesic medication. Such a drug can help the patient to cope with the symptoms, whether or not depression is present.

iii *Early morning awakening; difficulty in getting back to sleep:* This is one of the main symptoms of depression which, of course, can coexist with CFS or be a secondary 'reactive' response to the syndrome.

A thorough history will enable your GP to ascertain whether or not depression is a relevant factor in your pattern of sleep disturbance. If there are other symptoms that support this diagnosis, then it may be beneficial to try one of the tricyclic antidepressants at night. A small dose is often sufficient, but it can take up to a fortnight for the full benefits to become apparent. An additional sleeping pill is often unnecessary.

The benefits of a nightly dose of an antidepressant can therefore be twofold. It may help restore a normal sleeping pattern in those who are depressed by their CFS (and so make them feel better about their condition by day). And it is of enormous help in coping with the physical symptoms of CFS, which can last years and be devastating in the restrictions they impose upon the patient's lifestyle.

Tingling and numbness

Altered sensation is reported in over half of patients suffering CFS. This may take the form of paraesthesia (pins and needles), hypoaesthesia (numbness) or hyperaesthesia (increased sensitivity). The sensory nerves are affected and are involved in detecting changes in touch or sensation. This means that altered sensation may change the way we perceive pain, temperature and direct pressure to the skin surface.

The altered sensory perception is not always present. It fluctuates in severity and appears unrelated to external temperature changes. The hands and feet seem especially affected but any part of the body may be involved. Needless to say, patients should be aware of these changes in perception to avoid injury by burning or trauma. It can be very easy to misjudge the temperature of bath water or to be oblivious to cutting your finger with a sharp kitchen knife.

Other reasons for sensory nerve involvement should also be considered. These include multiple sclerosis, pernicious anaemia, diabetes, porphyria and vascular problems, some of which will be considered in more depth in Chapter 4.

Changes in mood

Mood changes affect nearly every patient with CFS. Depression is by far the most common. We have already looked at sleep disturbances in CFS, and one of the most frequent patterns corresponds with the sleep disturbance seen in depression. It is in those patients that an antidepressant is frequently of use. But this is not the case for every patient. There are many in whom an antidepressant would be useless.

In the early days of research into CFS it was thought that CFS was, in fact, a type of depression. More recent studies have shown the two conditions to be quite distinct, with laboratory findings proving it. If they coexist in some patients, then at least one aspect of their illness is amenable to treatment.

At the First World Congress on Chronic Fatigue Syndrome and Related Disorders, held in Brussels in November 1995, numerous studies were presented, reflecting the many aspects of CFS. Among them was a paper presented at the Neuropsychology session that suggested that CFS patients do not show a depressive attributional style (Dr A. S. Farmer, University of Wales College of Medicine). A double blind placebo-controlled trial of fluoxetine (Prozac) was described by Dr J. H. M. M. Vercoulen (University Hospital Nijmegen, the Netherlands). This involved two groups of patients—a depressed CFS group and a non-depressed CFS group. No beneficial effect on fatigue or any other dimension of CFS was observed after fluoxetine was given in a 20 mg daily dose.

Professor Anthony Komaroff (Professor of Medicine at Harvard University, Boston, USA) gave an address at the same congress, which he repeated nine days later in London. He gave three reasons for his belief that CFS and depression were separate illnesses. He spoke of a group of symptoms in CFS that did not reflect psychiatric illness. He also referred to a series of studies that found abnormalities in the hypothalamic-pituitary axis of the brain that were quite different from those found in patients with major depression. He emphasised that CFS failed to respond to psychiatric therapy (citing the studies with the antidepressant Prozac), and finally he drew attention to the absence of psychiatric disease in a large fraction of CFS patients, either before or after the onset of their illness.

The study of the hypothalamic-pituitary-adrenal axis mentioned by Professor Komaroff is of special interest. The hypothalamus makes hormones that affect the pituitary, and the pituitary makes hormones that affect the adrenal glands. In healthy people a normal amount is made by each of these glands. In major depression there is a very high amount of these chemicals made by each organ. But in CFS the very opposite occurs—an underproduction by the pituitary of ACTH (adreno-corticotrophic hormone), which leads to an underproduction of cortisol by the adrenal glands. This objective measure in CFS is different from healthy people, and even more so from those suffering major depression.

Depression occurs as a complicating condition in many illnesses. Heart attack and rheumatoid arthritis are two diverse examples. If, in addition, the central nervous system (CNS) is also affected by an illness, then the incidence of depression is even higher. The depression may represent an associated entity in these conditions, and not simply a reaction to the original illness. But in many such cases a reactive-type depression is the most common type to occur. CFS is a prime example, along with Parkinson's disease, epilepsy and multiple sclerosis.

Reactive depression is a depression for which there is good reason. As opposed to the deep-seated *endogenous depression*, where there are no obvious reasons why the patient should be depressed, a reactive depression usually has a very apparent cause or precipitating factor. If the cause of the depression is dealt with, the mood lifts and the depression is resolved.

Some of the more common symptoms of depression are mood changes, sleep disturbances, lack of libido and poor concentration. A wide gamut of emotions are involved apart from the obvious feeling 'low' or miserable. Frustration, anger, tearfulness and anxiety can all be found in patients who are depressed; and patients with CFS have good reason to feel all these emotions at various times during their protracted illness.

It is usual to see depression in patients who are suffering a loss. This may involve the loss of a loved one, a job, material things, self-esteem or one's health. In CFS the loss may be one or more of these. Indeed, if we are ill and cannot work there is a huge potential loss involving social, financial and emotional reasons. It is only by working through the illness, with the support of a network of doctor(s), family and friends that these losses may be reduced and the consequent depression minimised.

Fortunately, depression can be diagnosed and treated in most cases. It is one common consequence of CFS that does respond to therapy, whether that be of a supportive nature or using an antidepressant drug. The latter is of enormous value in many situations where some of the other features of CFS overlap with the depression—e.g. sleep disturbance, as discussed in (iii) above—although there are of course many situations where such medication is of no use at all.

Sleep disturbances, feeling miserable and coping with ongoing physical discomfort can all be improved with the judicious use of an antidepressant. Although the actual course of the illness will not be altered, the ability to cope with CFS may be improved enormously if depression co-exists. There are various types of antidepressant drugs. The tricyclic group is the most commonly prescribed, and I will discuss these in more detail in Chapter 5.

Secondary problems

Other problems faced by CFS patients include a wide range of symptoms, which may involve vision, hearing, joints, glands, the throat and the gastrointestinal system. Individually these affect far fewer patients than the main symptoms of muscle fatigue and brain malfunction. But their presence may lead to a complex clinical picture of which both patient and doctor should be aware. And, as already stated, the appearance of a new symptom may actually be unrelated to CFS and that possibility should always be taken into account.

Secondary symptoms and their treatment

Visual disturbances

i *Blurred vision:* The tiny eye (ciliary) muscles, like many others, can be affected by fatigue. Extended periods of reading, fine detailed work or watching a television or computer screen can cause these muscles to malfunction and can cause blurred vision, or even double vision. It is often shortlived and responds to rest.

ii *Photophobia:* An increased sensitivity to light can be caused by pupillary muscle malfunction. Sunlight, neon lights and other bright lighting can cause this symptom. Reducing the glare with dark glasses may help.

iii *Pain in the eye:* This is usually unilateral (affecting one eye), tends to occur behind the eye (retro-orbital pain), and responds to rest.

Auditory symptoms

Sound is transmitted through the external and middle ear where the waves cause vibration within the cochlea (a fluid-filled spiral chamber). Many tiny hairs within the cochlea transmit the sound into a nerve impulse, which is then transmitted to the brain via the auditory nerve. It is thought that in some CFS patients the conducting ability of the auditory nerve is disturbed. This causes:

i *Tinnitus:* a whistling, high-pitched, persistent sound that is distracting and distressing to the sufferer.

ii *Hyperacusis:* an abnormal acuteness of hearing leading to a painful sensitivity to noisy environments.

Tinnitus may be intermittent or self-limiting. If stress is a factor, as it can be, then treating the underlying cause is essential, with perhaps the short-term use of a tranquilliser. If the tinnitus is persistent, an ENT (ear, nose and throat) specialist's opinion should be sought and a masking device may be advised. Worn like a hearing-aid, this may disguise the sound and provide relief.

Arthralgia

Joint pain is reported in about a third of CFS sufferers. The pain is less severe than the more common muscle pain (myalgia) but may be related to the involvement of surrounding muscles and tendons. There are no permanent or degenerative changes in the joints, and a medical examination usually reveals no restriction of movements. Radiological (X-ray) examination is also normal.

Viral infections can cause a temporary arthritis, and we've already discussed the role of viruses in CFS. Fortunately viral arthritis tends to be self-limiting and the joint pains eventually subside.

More serious causes of joint pain must be excluded. Rheumatoid conditions and even simple osteoarthritis (following an old injury or repetitive use of the joint) can cause similar symptoms. But the absence of associated swelling is a clue to the benign nature of the arthralgia, as is the lack of deformity of the joint. X-rays and blood serology should exclude joint degeneration and rheumatoid disease.

All joint involvement in CFS is reversible and responds to simple treatment. If there is no contra-indication to their use, the non-steroidal anti-inflammatory drugs (including simple aspirin) should bring relief in most cases. And if the symptoms are less severe, evening primrose oil has been shown to have a good anti-inflammatory action.

Enlarged lymph glands

In the neck region (the submandibular and the parotid) enlarged lymph glands are frequently coupled with a sore throat and form the initial presenting clinical picture of many infections. Only a tiny proportion of such infections go on to become CFS. And the glandular enlargement in CFS may be intermittent or only very shortlived.

Most cases of lymphadenopathy (enlarged lymph nodes) are self-limiting. As a sign of infection, these nodes signal the body's immune response being 'turned on'. Most viral infections resolve and the bacterial infections usually respond to antibiotics, although the emergence in recent years of antibiotic-resistant strains has become a major concern. Throat swabs and blood tests may be required and are necessary to diagnose conditions like infectious mono-nucleosis (glandular fever), which may last for months.

Persistent lymphadenopathy is an indication of a more serious illness in most cases. A thorough history and physical examination may lead a doctor to suspect a leukaemia or a cancer with lymphatic involvement. Blood tests and lymph node biopsies will be required in such cases, with further investigations performed according to the patient's symptomatology.

Irritable bowel syndrome (IBS)

This is a group of symptoms affecting the gastrointestinal tract and occurs in up to 15 per cent of the general population. The incidence is thought to be approximately twice that among CFS sufferers.

There is almost certainly a multifactoral basis for IBS. We have already discussed the role of the autonomic nervous system and its supply to the gut wall earlier in this chapter. And some patients, both with and without CFS, may go on to develop IBS following a gastrointestinal infection (e.g. food poisoning or a gastric virus). In other patients, symptoms can be aggravated or perpetuated by certain foods. And, as in so many conditions, stress/anxiety is a significant factor in the aetiology of IBS.

The main symptoms of IBS are abdominal discomfort, bloatedness, nausea and a change in bowel habit. The pain is frequently colicky (waxing and waning) in nature and is relieved by a bowel motion. The bloatedness or abdominal distension is due to the excessive production of wind or flatulence and can certainly be aggravated by certain foods. And the change in bowel habit can be anything from sluggish bowels and constipation to loose stools and diarrhoea.

Investigation of the symptoms of IBS usually fails to show any major abnormality. Stool cultures should be performed in the case of persistent diarrhoea to exclude other causes of a potentially treatable nature (e.g. infections such as giardia). Sigmoidoscopy (endoscopic examination of the distal part of the large bowel) should be performed to exclude more sinister causes of change in bowel habit (e.g. carcinoma, ulcerative colitis), and is essentially normal in patients with IBS. Other causes of abdominal pain (e.g. gastric and duodenal ulcers, gall stones and cholecystitis) should also be excluded by a gastroscopy/duodenoscopy or by radiography. If there is still a doubt about the diagnosis, then scanning by ultrasound or CAT scan may be necessary.

Treatment of IBS is directed largely at the symptoms. Abdominal pain may respond to antispasmodic drugs (mebeverine hydrochloride or Colofac, dicyclomine hydrochloride or Merbentyl) and dietary modification (see Chapter 5). Constipation should be treated with an increased amount of dietary fibre (both granular and cellular fibre) and a good fluid intake. Laxatives are seldom required and should be avoided. The other extreme, where loose stools are a problem, will respond to a carefully introduced regimen of codeine phosphate (15–30 mg) up to three or four times a day if necessary. Stress management is also worthwhile to prevent exacerbations of IBS, and is also advisable in managing the total picture of CFS. This will be discussed in detail in Chapter 5.

Irritable bowel syndrome will usually respond very favourably to the diet recommended in Chapter 5. Those dietary principles help many other aspects of CFS as well, and I cannot overemphasise their importance. So many of the illnesses and diseases we face today can be prevented by a good diet and lifestyle. The diet I recommend will also help prevent cardiovascular disease, diverticular disease, diabetes, many types of cancer as well as degenerative joint disease.

Weight changes

Patients with CFS have a tendency to put on weight and therefore have an increased risk of allied health problems (e.g. hypertension or high blood pressure, diabetes). This is primarily due to their enforced immobility rather than to any metabolic or glandular disorder, although eminently treatable conditions like hypothyroidism should be excluded as part of the screening process. The generally inactive lifestyle imposed upon CFS patients means that their caloric requirements are usually less than those of a healthy person. In addition, the frequent feelings of fatigue tend to make patients want to eat; we tend to equate food with energy, and it takes great will-power to accept that increased caloric input does not solve the problem in CFS.

One group of CFS patients can actually suffer weight loss. These are usually the younger group who are actively growing while fighting the debilitating symptoms of CFS. Children have more difficulty in regaining weight and can become almost anorexic if their diet is not carefully supervised. Their special needs are discussed in Chapter 7.

I have often found in practice that a calorie-controlled diet is usually much healthier and more balanced than a non-restrictive diet. This is because one must think of how to get the most nutritional value and balance for a limited number of calories. A good dietary plan is essential, not only for sufferers of CFS, but to maintain good health and prevent other disorders which are so prevalent in the wider community. By adhering to the dietary principles laid down in Chapter 5, calories should not be a problem.

Summary

Chronic fatigue syndrome is defined by:

persistent, relapsing chronic fatigue that is not the result of ongoing exertion and which results in substantial reduction in occupational, social and personal activities;

four or more of the following symptoms that are present for six months or more and which do not pre-date the fatigue:
- impaired short-term memory or concentration
- sore throat with associated lymphadenopathy
- myalgia
- arthralgia
- headaches
- sleep disturbance
- post-exertional malaise lasting more than 24 hours.

The following are the main features of chronic fatigue syndrome and their approximate frequencies in patients:

Muscle fatigue, 100 per cent
Brain malfunction, demonstrated by
- impaired short-term memory or concentration, 80 per cent
- headaches, 75 per cent
- autonomic-related symptoms; 70 per cent have at least one of these:
  - heart- and blood vessel-related symptoms
  - temperature regulation disturbance
  - irritable bowel syndrome
  - bladder dysfunction
  - micturition syncope
- balance disturbance, 75 per cent
- sleep disturbance, 66 per cent
- tingling and numbness, 55 per cent
- changes in mood, 90 per cent

Secondary problems; less than 50 per cent:
- visual disturbances
- auditory symptoms
- arthralgia
- enlarged lymph nodes
- irritable bowel syndrome
- weight changes.

Chapter four

Diagnosis of CFS

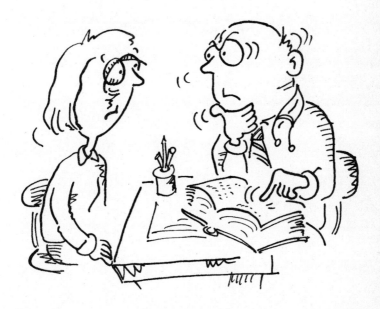

Due to the wide range of symptoms involved, CFS does not affect everyone in the same way. While fatigue is common to all patients, the other prominent symptoms discussed in Chapter 3 differ from patient to patient, both in their frequency and severity.

The onset of CFS can be either acute or more gradual. Approximately 40 per cent of patients can recall a specific viral-type illness from which they did not fully recover. They describe their symptoms as starting from that point in time. A further 30 per cent of patients talk about a more insidious onset of the illness. This group reports a gradually increasing tiredness that is combined with the symptoms of muscle fatigue and brain malfunction of varying degree. The remaining 30 per cent give a history suggesting an infectious cause to their illness that was not especially acute or obvious to start with.

Adult acute onset

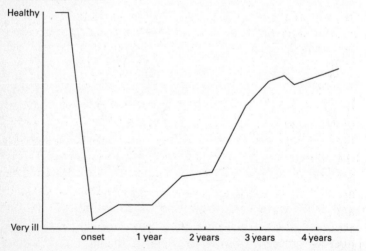

Figure 4.1 The most common course of CFS in adults, with an acute flu-like onset, followed by slow and steady recovery over several years. From Bell, D. S., *The Doctor's Guide to Chronic Fatigue Syndrome*, p. 139, Addison-Wesley Publishing Company, 1993, 1994. Copyright © 1994, 1995 by David S. Bell MD.

Adult gradual onset

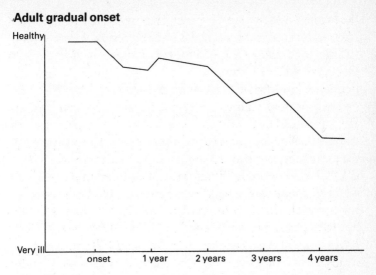

Figure 4.2 Gradual onset of CFS with prolonged course over years. Patients with this type of onset seem to be less ill than those with acute onset, but also seem to have less chance of complete recovery. This pattern is more common in younger children. From Bell, D. S., *The Doctor's Guide to Chronic Fatigue Syndrome*, p. 139, Addison-Wesley Publishing Company, 1993, 1994. Copyright © 1994, 1995 by David S. Bell MD.

In the case of the younger patient it is important to be aware of these differences in onset. The majority of adolescent patients with CFS present with an acute onset illness, while the younger child (under ten years) will usually have a more gradual or insidious onset of symptoms. Younger children are at a disadvantage in that they are less able to recognise and describe the cognitive aspects of their illness. As a consequence they have been frequently misdiagnosed in the past as suffering from a variety of ailments, ranging from attention deficit disorder to rheumatoid arthritis and school phobias.

With an illness of such varying symptoms and onset it is little wonder that both the medical profession and the general public are so bewildered by the term 'chronic fatigue syndrome'. Many doctors feel threatened by a disorder for which there are few clear-cut parameters. There are no specific tests to confirm CFS, its aetiology is still unclear and, until we know more about it, a cure or specific treatment is unlikely to be discovered.

Conventional medical teaching tends to concentrate on the illnesses with which we are familiar. It does not always prepare us for those situations where, quite frankly, we have not got much to offer. Many doctors like to appear infallible. They do not feel 'in control' where a patient presents with symptoms for which they do not have all the answers. It is therefore no surprise that patients have turned increasingly to alternative medicine in recent years.

Most doctors accept that CFS does exist. How else could one explain why a number of patients in their prime (mostly in their thirties and forties), and with no significant past medical history, are struck by an illness which by its very nature prevents them from continuing their normal and busy lives? I have already said that the term 'yuppie flu' is neither accurate nor appropriate. However, what it may imply is that most CFS sufferers are people in their prime and usually high achievers—the last group one could imagine being labelled 'malingerers' or 'hysterics'.

It is an unfortunate fact that a significant minority of the medical profession are ill-equipped to treat patients with CFS. They see the disorder as a 'waste-basket' diagnosis. The very name implies (unfortunately) that it is an illness of a somewhat trivial nature. It is a prolonged disorder, with relapses and remissions, and has a neuropsychiatric component, as well as the fatigue. Its acceptance as an organic disorder rather than a psychiatric one has not been without controversy. Yet, despite the scientific advances that are being made in relation to CFS, there are still sceptics who see medicine as black and white, with no shades of grey.

Once a diagnosis of CFS has been made it is imperative that the patient has confidence and trust in the doctor. If the doctor is knowledgeable about CFS and is abreast of current thinking, then, providing a rapport exists, the doctor will be able to help the patient manage and cope with the illness over a period which may extend to at least several years. On the other hand, if the doctor is ignorant about CFS, has doubts about its existence or sees it as a psychiatric condition, then the patient must go elsewhere for help.

There are many doctors today who are up to date and who can accept the fact that there are conditions they must treat without all the answers being given in the textbooks or journals. If doctors confined their practice to only those clearly recognisable disorders, then medicine would be a very restrictive profession indeed.

Pinpointing the disease

Fatigue is a common symptom of many different conditions. If one were to examine the list of patients seen by a GP at the end of the day it is likely that a good many would have listed being 'tired' as one of their complaints.

As in most medical conditions, the history-taking is important. Fatigue is usually just one of a number of symptoms, all of which tend to come together and suggest a diagnosis or a 'short list' of differential diagnoses.

During the history-taking the doctor may well have noted certain characteristics about the fatigue. Further questioning of the patient should reveal the nature of the fatigue, its duration, the things that make it better or worse and the other symptoms with which it is associated. The patient's occupation, family life and social activities are also important in obtaining an accurate history.

The history should be followed by a physical examination. The extent of the examination will depend on the symptoms volunteered by the patient and any further areas suspected by the doctor. Complete physical examinations may be indicated in certain situations; for example where a systemic condition is involved. In a more straightforward case, where the diagnosis is simple and localised, the examination is brief and directed at a specific problem. For example, following a ten-day history of sore throat, fever and tiredness, an examination of the throat may reveal enlarged, inflamed tonsils. The ears should also be checked and certainly the regional glands will be palpated. The diagnosis of tonsillitis is most probable, but if glandular fever is suspected the doctor may feel for other enlarged glands and an enlarged spleen. He or she may decide to take a blood sample to confirm or exclude glandular fever, and/or a throat swab to identify the infective organism.

Where fatigue has been prolonged, relapsing, not the result of ongoing exertion but aggravated by exertion nevertheless, the doctor may concentrate on the cause of the fatigue. Associated symptoms obtained from a thorough history will help to define the problem. But if a physical examination is essentially normal, then a diagnostic problem arises. It is at this point that a list of differential diagnoses must be considered. And the question of specific screening tests arises.

The list of symptoms we examined in the previous chapter shows what a wide-ranging number of conditions can be suggested by a patient with CFS. These may well be conditions that are quite treatable and will respond dramatically to the correct measures. So it is important to consider, and exclude, a large number of illnesses early in the patient's management.

Other conditions that may present with chronic fatigue can be categorised as follows:

Infectious
- Viral
- Tuberculosis
- Lyme disease
- Q fever
- Brucellosis
- Toxoplasmosis

Rheumatic
- Fibromyalgia

- Rheumatoid arthritis
- Sjogren's syndrome
- Systemic lupus erythematosis (SLE)

Neurological
- Multiple sclerosis
- Parkinson's disease

Glandular/Hormonal
- Hypothyroidism
- Hyperthyroidism
- Addison's disease

Depression

Miscellaneous
- Myasthenia gravis
- Anaemia
- Hodgkin's disease
- Chronic ciguatera poisoning
- Alcoholism
- Hypercalcaemia
- 'Sick building' syndrome
- Neoplasm (malignancy)

Infectious

We have already examined the role of **viruses** in CFS in Chapter 2. Needless to say, the proportion of viral illnesses that trigger the abnormal immune response thought to be responsible for CFS is very much a minority. However, viral illnesses are common in the community, and they have become an increasingly important field for researchers in recent years with the growing threat of HIV infection (and AIDS), new strains of hepatitis and a possible role in carcinogenesis.

Most of the common viral infections seen in general practice can cause a 'post-viral fatigue'. A significant percentage of influenza victims will be unwell for several weeks or even months, with muscle aches and fatigue. And the devastating picture seen in young patients with glandular fever can mimic CFS. Caused by the Epstein-Barr virus, glandular fever can last for many months and tends to occur in teenagers during their final years at school. Most GPs will have found profound fatigue, sore throat and swollen glands suffered by these younger patients, who may be forced to repeat a year at school or university due to their illness. It is essential that they have enforced rest and that their progress is monitored with regular blood tests every two or three weeks to measure atypical lymphocytes (white blood cells). And of course the specific infectious mononucleosis test for glandular fever is positive, although it may take several weeks into the illness before becoming so.

HIV infection can present in many different ways. It is always important to remember that lymphadenopathy (swollen glands), unexplained fever, memory or concentration difficulties, and marked fatigue are some of them. In developed nations most patients at risk of HIV infection are aware of the consequences. Unfortunately that is not the case elsewhere and the number of AIDS cases is increasing at an alarming rate.

If a patient suspects that he or she may have come in contact with the AIDS virus, it is essential to be tested. Most cases are still transmitted by sexual contact (blood, semen, body fluids) and especially by gay sex. But needle-stick injuries, blood transfusions and intravenous drug use are other means by which the virus may be spread. Allowing for a three-month period to sero-convert, a simple blood test will reveal whether you are HIV positive. This can be organised by your GP or, if you wish, through one of the many clinics set up for the treatment of sexually transmitted diseases.

Infections of a non-viral nature can also cause fatigue. It is alarming that, as we reach the year 2000, there is an upswing in the incidence of **tuberculosis** in Australia. Some cases have been the result of inadequate screening of new migrants to the country. In addition to fatigue, the patient will suffer weight loss and recurring fever. Chest X-ray and sputum cultures will confirm the diagnosis and, unlike most viral infections, the tuberculosis is responsive to chemotherapy (usually triple therapy).

Lyme disease is transmitted by tick bites. Apart from fatigue, the symptoms include a characteristic circular rash, joint and muscle pains, and facial nerve paralysis. A blood test will confirm the diagnosis and, fortunately, the infection responds to antibiotics.

Q fever is caused by a small intracellular bacterium (*Coxiella burnettii*), which is usually found in the dust after having spread from slaughtered infected animals. It is seen mostly in abattoir workers. The dominant symptoms are headaches, nausea, night sweats, myalgia and an incapacitating fatigue. About 20 per cent of cases progress to a 'post-Q fever syndrome', which is virtually identical to CFS. This can be prevented by the use of doxycycline (an antibiotic) in the acute stage of the illness.

Q fever is an important occupational hazard for workers in the meat and livestock industry. About 1000 cases are reported in Australia each year. Diagnosis in the acute stage is dependent upon the patient's symptomatology, as serum antibody tests are not distinctive at this stage. The advantage of early diagnosis is obvious.

Other infections related to farm animals include **brucellosis** (from unpasteurised milk) and **toxoplasmosis** (from undercooked meat). Both can cause flu-like illnesses, with the latter producing an almost identical picture to glandular fever. And both can be diagnosed by specific blood tests.

Rheumatic

Fibromyalgia syndrome

Fibromyalgia syndrome is the current terminology for a long-recognised condition characterised by musculoskeletal pain (generalised or regional) and abnormal areas of soft-tissue tenderness ('tender points'). The pain is usually chronic and varies in severity, but it can be serious enough to disrupt every aspect of the patient's life. The perception of pain is affected and pain threshold tends to be low.

Fibromyalgia syndrome affects about 4 per cent of the population and in the past has had several other labels, including 'soft-tissue rheumatism' and the inaccurate 'fibrositis' (where the '-itis' implies inflammation, which may not in fact be present). Females outnumber males in a ratio of about six-to-one with a peak prevalence in the thirties and forties age groups, which is similar to CFS. Like CFS, it can affect any socio-economic group, and is frequently associated with other ancillary disorders.

There are various other symptoms, including fatigue that can be so prominent as to become the main symptom. Other common findings are abnormal sensations (peripheral numbness), sleep disturbances (specifically a lack of non-REM sleep), psychological distress, and joint stiffness (especially in the mornings). Tension-type headaches are common and feelings of swelling can also occur in more than half the cases, with occasional cyclical oedema and mastalgia reported.

Less common symptoms include Raynaud's phenomenon, where cold hands and feet result from a vascular system overreacting to changes in temperature. Symptoms of both irritable bowel syndrome and irritable bladder syndrome may also be noticed, the latter causing an 'interstitial cystitis' (bladder infection).

Both the pain and the fatigue can be aggravated by certain factors. Weather change is particularly relevant, with patients often predicting a change in climate before it actually occurs. Physical activity and mental stress are also known to exacerbate the condition.

Disability may affect every aspect of a patient's life. Recreational pursuits and household tasks need to be modified frequently and work activities may be severely curtailed.

Diagnosis of the fibromyalgia syndrome relies on both the history of symptoms and the finding of widespread tender points. The American College of Rheumatology criteria suggest an 85 per cent specificity and sensitivity for this disorder if (a) eleven out of eighteen predesignated sites are abnormally tender, and (b) there is widespread pain above and below the diaphragm on both sides of the body.

There are no specific investigations, as diagnosis is based on clinical findings. But a full-blood examination (FBE) and erythrocyte sedimentation rate (ESR) are advisable, together with a serology test for rheumatoid factor, antinuclear antibody and a creatinine kinase level. Other biochemical tests may be necessary (including thyroid function) depending on the patient's presenting features.

Although there is no specific or effective treatment for fibromyalgia, a number of approaches may be of benefit. Physiotherapy, Tai Chi exercises, yoga and the Feldenkraus technique are often helpful. The latter involves re-educating motion patterns to make a patient more aware of pain-related movements. A graded aerobic program is advisable, and the use of low-dose tricyclic antidepressants may help the sleep pattern, along with basic sleep hygiene (see Chapter 7). Occasional injections of steroids into the tender spots may be required, but simple non-narcotic analgesics are often enough. Relaxation techniques and long-term coping strategies are also an important aspect of management.

Rheumatoid arthritis

This is a very chronic generalised condition affecting mainly the more peripheral joints. It is characterised by swelling of the synovial (lining) membranes of the joints and the surrounding tissues, with associated generalised symptoms of malaise, fatigue and peripheral paraesthesia. There is subchondral osteoporosis (thinning and rarefaction of bone) and, in advanced stages, there may be erosion of cartilage and bone with wasting of the associated muscles. These latter changes give rise to the characteristic deviations and deformity of this severe disorder.

The disease can occur at all ages but it is most common in middle age. Females are affected at least twice as often as males, and there is frequently a family history of the disorder. There is also an autoimmune element to the disease, whereby an abnormal immune response occurs to a component of the body's own tissues. The presence of abnormal antibodies in the serum is one of its distinguishing diagnostic features.

In most cases the onset is insidious, with fatigue and general malaise accompanying the transient joint and muscular pain. The small joints of the hands and feet are the first to become involved, but as the disease progresses it may spread to involve the wrists, elbows, ankles, shoulders and knees, with the hips involved in only the most severe cases. In about 10 per cent of patients the onset is more acute, with low-grade fever, rapid heart beat (tachycardia) and joint involvement.

The muscles are involved from the outset of the disease. Muscular stiffness is a prominent early symptom. It is especially marked in the mornings or after a period of inactivity. Muscular atrophy (wasting) is also a frequent finding. Spasm of the muscles can also give rise to flexion deformities, which may be correctable in the early stages. But in advanced disease, contractures will become permanent, with characteristic deformity of the hands and finger joints.

The early phases of rheumatoid arthritis are characterised by remissions and relapses. X-rays of affected joints will show demineralisation, or thinning, of the bone ends. As the disease advances, the characteristic narrowing of joint spaces will occur, with marginal erosions and eventual deformity of the joints.

Subcutaneous nodules are found in a significant proportion of patients. These are often found on the forearms below the elbow joints and may also occur over the fingers, kneecaps, sacrum and scalp. Other less common connective tissue abnormalities can occur in the later stages of the disease, giving rise to a diverse range of symptoms including purpura, bruising, leg ulcers, pericarditis and pleurisy.

Diagnosis of rheumatoid arthritis is not difficult in the later stages, with characteristic symptoms and deformities. The radiological changes mentioned above also aid the diagnosis. But in the early stages it may be confused with a great many other conditions including CFS, osteoarthritis, gout, rheumatic fever and rarer forms of arthritis.

Blood tests are extremely valuable. In particular, the specific rheumatoid factor test is positive, along with the demonstration of increased antibody levels, a raised ESR and possibly a hypochromic (low haemoglobin) anaemia and mild polymorph leucocytosis (increased white cell count).

The treatment of rheumatoid arthritis is largely symptomatic. Bed rest is advised in the acute phase where there is fever, swollen and painful joints, and a raised ESR. Anti-inflammatory drugs have been used with success for many years, as have corticosteroid drugs, which can bring dramatic relief but must be used with great caution.

Physiotherapy and hydrotherapy are both essential after the acute phase of the illness, and help in maintaining joint mobility. In some patients, gold injections have their place, but they must be controlled and monitored closely. Toxic reaction may occur and blood and urine tests must be performed regularly.

Sjogren's syndrome

Sjogren's syndrome is a rarer disease in which fatigue is accompanied by polyarthritis. Like rheumatoid arthritis and systemic lupus erythematosis (SLE), it is also thought to be an autoimmune disorder. It is characterised by dryness of the eyes and mouth due to reduction in the secretion of tears and diminished secretion by the mucous glands of the upper respiratory and gastrointestinal tracts. Keratoconjunctivitis and the presence of corneal ulceration are diagnostic.

Treatment is essentially the same as that recommended for rheumatoid arthritis. In addition, local inflammation of the eyes is controlled by hydrocortisone eye drops and hypromellose drops to provide lubrication.

Systemic lupus erythematosis (SLE)

This is a rare but diffuse disorder involving connective tissue. The disorder is more common in young women and, unlike Sjogren's syndrome, the symptoms are varied. In addition to fatigue, muscle pain and joint involvement, patients commonly present with fever and an acute erythematous eruption on the face, with the cheeks showing a characteristic 'butterfly' distribution.

Other symptoms are diverse and include weight loss, anorexia, pleural effusion, pericarditis, pneumonitis, and diffuse or local alopecia (hair loss). Raynaud's phenomenon (cold hands and feet) and various neurological symptoms may also make the diagnosis difficult in the early stages.

SLE is diagnosed by the demonstration of an antibody to nuclear material. This is present in the majority of cases and puts SLE in the group of autoimmune disorders with rheumatoid arthritis and Sjogren's syndrome.

Corticosteroids are the treatment of choice in the acute stages of SLE. Longer-term therapies include chloroquine, which is especially useful in controlling skin lesions.

Neurological diseases

Multiple sclerosis

Multiple sclerosis (MS) is the most likely neurological condition to be confused with CFS. It affects people in the same major age group (20–50) with maximum incidence among young adults. The course of the illness is relapsing and remitting, with multiple symptomatology reflecting the widely scattered lesions.

Multiple sclerosis is due to the destruction of the myelin sheaths that surround the nerve fibres in the white matter of the brain, the spinal cord and the optic nerves. The cause is not known but, as with CFS, there are thought to be trigger factors which include trauma, infection and allergy.

Fatigue is common to both multiple sclerosis and CFS and is worse after exertion and in extremes of temperature. The other shared symptoms include problems with balance and altered skin sensations. Mood changes and visual disturbances can also occur in both, with one very important exception.

Retrobulbar neuritis is specific to multiple sclerosis and is the most frequent presenting symptom in younger patients. In those over 50, it is weakness of one or both lower limbs that presents first, as a result of corticospinal tract demyelination, which can develop suddenly. The effect may be very slight with little disability, or it can be quite crippling.

Brainstem and cerebellar demyelination produce a further range of symptoms, which are beyond the scope of this book. Suffice to say that the early symptoms of multiple sclerosis and those of CFS may be very similar indeed. Especially the weakness of limbs, the balance problems and the fatigue.

Diagnosis of multiple sclerosis is usually made by a thorough neurological examination. Pallor of the temporal half of one or both optic discs is common, even without visual symptoms. Nystagmus (an involuntary rapid movement of the eyeball), intention tremor, abnormal reflexes and altered muscle tone are also found.

Abnormalities of the cerebrospinal fluid (obtained by lumbar puncture) will suggest the diagnosis. An abnormal proportion of proteins is found, together with a mild lymphocytosis (excessive number of lymphocytes). Magnetic resonance imaging (MRI) will confirm the characteristic brain lesions that result from the destruction of tissue and the presence of glial scarring.

Parkinson's disease

This neurological condition, resulting from damage to the basal ganglia in the brain, also needs to be considered. The earliest stages may overlap somewhat with CFS (muscle pain, visual symptoms and muscle fasciculation). But the development of the characteristic muscle rigidity, the marked rhythmical tremor and the hypokinesis (decreased mobility) of Parkinsonism soon become so obvious that the diagnosis is unlikely to be mistaken.

Glandular/Hormonal disorders

Among this group of disorders, the most important are disorders of the thyroid glands which must be excluded. They are fairly easily diagnosed clinically and can be confirmed by a simple blood test.

Hypothyroidism

An underactive thyroid gland leads to a variety of symptoms. In addition to marked fatigue, the patient will also be sensitive to cold, have a dry (and possibly lemon-tinted) skin, and hoarseness, weight gain, loss of hair and maybe swelling of the tissues (especially the eyelids). If there is swelling (or oedema), the condition is known as 'myxoedema'.

The symptoms are the result of lowered metabolism and slowing of both physical and mental activity. A physical examination is often diagnostic, with swollen face, puffy eyelids, rough skin and hair loss. The patient speaks with a slow, monotonous voice that is frequently hoarse. Mental impairment is often obvious, with the lethargic patient having a poor memory and a slowed reaction time.

Changes are often apparent on the electrocardiogram (myocardial ischaemia) and chest X-ray (an enlarged heart shadow). But the definitive test is a measure of thyroid hormones in the blood.

Treatment usually involves the use of thyroxine, which must be maintained indefinitely. Periodic blood tests are required to check the level of thyroid function.

Hyperthyroidism

Hyperthyroidism condition results from the excessive production and secretion of thyroid hormone. It is much more common in women and usually occurs in early adult life.

The symptoms include many of those seen in anxiety states. Nervousness, restlessness, tremor, tachycardia and palpitations are all presented, combined with an intolerance of heat, muscle weakness, fatigue, and frequently loss of weight. The muscle weakness often resembles that seen in myasthenia gravis (see below).

Physical examination may reveal an enlarged thyroid gland (goitre) and a rather typical increased prominence of the eyes due to both lid-retraction and exophthalmos (where the eye is pushed forward in the orbital cavity due to swelling of the tissues behind the eye). A raised pulse rate and possibly extrasystoles (extra heart beats) may be found, with clammy skin and obvious weight loss, despite an often increased appetite. The latter is due to the increased body metabolism, which occurs with an excessive amount of circulating thyroxine.

Treatment is most frequently non-surgical, although partial thyroidectomy may be required if an enlarged thyroid does not respond adequately to antithyroid drugs and is obstructing the airway. Antithyroid drugs (such as carbimazole or propylthiouracil) suppress the secretion of thyroid hormones. But the dosage must be carefully monitored to avoid toxic effects such as granulocytosis (a blood disorder where a decreased number of white blood cells are manufactured, leading to a severe ulcerative condition of the throat and mucous membranes).

Addison's disease

This rare condition is due to a deficiency of the adrenocortical hormones (including cortisol). It occurs when the adrenal glands (which are located near the kidneys) are removed or destroyed by disease, such as tuberculosis, amyloidosis or carcinomatous metastatic deposits (advanced cancer).

Symptoms include muscle weakness and fatigue, loss of weight, low blood pressure, and gastrointestinal symptoms (including nausea, vomiting and diarrhoea). There is also a rather characteristic brownish skin pigmentation, which is due to an excessive production of melanocyte-stimulating hormone by the pituitary gland.

Diagnosis can be made by blood tests. The treatment is simply cortisone replacement therapy, assuming that no sinister underlying pathology is affecting the adrenal glands.

Depression

It is an unfortunate fact that some doctors who are unfamiliar with CFS are still misdiagnosing the condition as a 'type of depression'. There is no question that secondary depression can be a very real consequence of CFS, but the illness itself is definitely not a psychiatric disorder.

It is not difficult, however, to see why the two conditions could be confused in certain cases. Nearly half of all patients suffering from depression first present to their doctor with complaints that suggest physical illness. Although depression has its own very specific symptoms (see below), they may be overlooked or not elicited from the history.

Unfortunately, many general practitioners tend to be overbooked and overburdened. When they are trying to see a large number of patients in too short a time the physical symptoms with which the patient presents may lead them down the wrong path. All too often the leading questions that would uncover a depressive condition are not asked, and the patient is sent off with the wrong diagnosis. Fruitless investigations may be performed—few of which would be necessary if a thorough history had first been obtained.

Some of the common *physical* complaints that are made by a patient suffering from depression include fatigue, headaches, muscular aches and pains, gastrointestinal symptoms (including nausea, abdominal pain and constipation), dryness of the mouth, difficulty breathing and menstrual disturbances.

These 'physical' symptoms are mediated through the autonomic nervous system, and caused by changes in bodily functions associated with depression. We have already discussed the role of the autonomic nervous system in Chapter 3, so the similarity is obvious. Apart from fatigue, which is always present, two or three of the following symptoms are almost invariably present to some degree in most patients suffering from CFS.

The line of questioning to determine whether the problem is primarily a depressive illness is to ask about the specific symptoms of depression. These are:

- *Mood change:* The most fundamental abnormality in depressed patients, the mood can vary from mild despondency to overwhelming despair.
- *Loss of interest:* This may involve work, hobbies, home duties, personal appearance and libido. Patients do not always volunteer this information, but it must be discussed.
- *Sleep disturbances:* Difficulty getting to sleep, abnormal dreams, and especially early morning awakening are frequent symptoms of depression.
- *Difficulty in concentrating:* Simple tasks like reading and watching television become an effort. Decision making and conversation with others are also a problem for many depressed patients.
- *Self-doubts/Paranoia:* The depressed patient becomes preoccupied with himself or herself. They tend to magnify problems and then blame themselves for creating the dilemma. They have few bright thoughts and the whole

atmosphere becomes one of pessimism. He or she may occasionally be paranoid and suspect that people are against them.

- *Suicidal thoughts:* All depressed patients need to be asked whether they have ever felt suicidal. Because of their mood changes they are certainly at increased risk (especially males).

- *Anxiety:* This accompanies many illnesses and affects most of the population at some time or other. It can be persistent in depressed patients and, combined with restlessness, causes them to become agitated. In its severe form it may need treating in addition to the underlying depression.

- *Hypochondriasis:* Patients can become introverted and especially concerned over their own health. Relatively minor symptoms can assume greater importance than they deserve.

- *Irritability:* Depressed patients tend to be excessively irritable and difficult to live with. This is most obvious in the home situation.

- *Physical retardation:* In severe cases of depression the patients slow up in their movements and become almost stuporous.

That the patient is depressed may be clinically obvious. The furrowed brow, down-turned mouth and immobile expression can be immediately recognised. Stooped posture, slowed motor movements or restless agitation may also be apparent before he or she starts to speak.

In primary depression the predominant feature is persisting mood change. Onset is usually gradual and the length of the illness can vary greatly. All ages are affected, with women outnumbering men.

Precipitating factors are relevant in depressed patients. The illness is especially likely to occur following:

- physical illness, especially chronic conditions (e.g. CFS)
- bereavement
- pregnancy and parturition (giving birth).

For many years, depression was categorised as being endogenous (or severe), reactive (or mild), or a combination of both.

In the **endogenous** type the symptoms are more severe. There is a genetic element, and the onset may well have been independent of adverse environmental changes. Symptoms are worse in the morning, improving later in the day. Loss of weight and poor libido can be marked, together with early morning awakening. Interestingly, the depressed mood is *not* altered by improving environmental surroundings.

In the more common **reactive** depression the patient is more likely to be reacting to unfavourable circumstances or the loss of something (e.g. loved one, job, health, self-esteem). Symptoms are usually milder, with anxiety and sleep disturbance quite prominent. Patients tend to be younger than in the endogenous group and many improve once the precipitating factor is identified and remedied. It is this type of depression that is most likely to occur as a secondary symptom in CFS.

Treatment of depression has improved in recent decades. A large number of patients with reactive depression can be helped by psychotherapy alone. Some need antidepressants, and these have improved both in efficiency and tolerability over the years. A low dose of a tricyclic antidepressant given at night may control the symptoms during the course of the illness and is especially useful in the presence of chronic physical symptoms (e.g. CFS, rheumatoid arthritis).

The more severe type of depression is more resistant to treatment. Psychotherapy is seldom useful. In the past, electroconvulsive therapy (ECT) was especially effective in endogenous depression, but it has largely been superseded by the wide range of drugs available today.

Miscellaneous disorders

Myasthenia gravis

Myasthenia gravis is characterised by abnormal fatigue of certain muscles with an incapacity to sustain muscular activity. It is thought to be linked with an abnormal immune system, and is sometimes associated with thyrotoxicosis (where the thyroid gland is overactive), Hashimoto's disease (a type of thyroiditis), rheumatoid arthritis and pernicious anaemia.

The disorder occurs more often in females than males, and young adults are the group most affected. It tends to run a remitting course, with relapses precipitated by physical and mental stress, including pregnancy.

The predominant symptom is a painless weakness of the muscles. This is worse later in the day and starts by affecting the facial muscles first. As a result, the early signs include intermittent ptosis (due to drooping of the upper eyelid muscle) and diplopia (double vision). The limb muscles become involved, making the most trivial tasks almost impossible. Also affected are the muscles used to chew, swallow, speak and breathe. Indeed, if the intercostal (chest) muscles are involved the patient could die of respiratory failure.

In the absence of other physical signs, the diagnosis is made on the presence of characteristic fatiguability of muscles. The immediate response to an intramuscular injection of neostigmine is also a diagnostic aid. Neostigmine was the mainstay of treatment, given in conjunction with atropine to diminish any undesirable side-effects of neostigmine such as bowel colic. Pyridostigmine (Mestinon) has a more prolonged action with fewer side-effects.

Anaemia

Iron-deficiency anaemia is by far the most common and should be fairly easy to diagnose. Symptoms of tiredness and fatigue may be associated with a poor diet or possibly bleeding (e.g. heavy menstrual blood loss). The patient is usually pale, with glossitis, stomatitis and conjunctival pallor. More sinister causes include occult blood loss from the gastrointestinal tract (e.g. ulcer, malignancy) and chronic infections.

Pernicious anaemia damages the nerves in the spinal cord and, in addition to the symptoms above, causes pins and needles (paraesthesia). Middle-aged females are the group most affected and the condition is often familial. An absence of gastric acid prevents the gastric mucosa from producing an intrinsic factor, which is required for the absorption of vitamin B12 from the alimentary tract.

Anaemia is confirmed by a blood examination. This reveals a low level of haemoglobin (the oxygen-carrying pigment of the red blood cell) and red blood cells, which have a reduced diameter (microcytosis) in iron-deficiency states. In other anaemias (including pernicious), the diameter of the red cells may actually be greater than normal (macrocytosis) together with other cell abnormalities. If pernicious anaemia is suspected, the blood levels of vitamin B12 and folate should also be measured. As anaemias may indicate the presence of more serious illnesses, other more specialised investigations may be indicated.

Treatment of uncomplicated chronic anaemias is quite straightforward. In nutritional iron-deficiency anaemia an appropriate diet rich in iron is required (red meat, leafy green vegetables), with possible iron supplementation (Fergon, Ferrogradumet). Patients with pernicious anaemia will require hydroxocobalamin injections (Neo-cytamen) to replace the vitamin B12 they cannot absorb.

Needless to say, if the anaemia is associated with a more serious underlying illness then that must be treated on its own merits. Anaemias are often associated with conditions as diverse as rheumatoid arthritis, chronic renal (and other) infections, and malignant disease. It is important that you note any unusual symptoms and report them to your GP. Only your symptoms and your doctor's examination for evidence of vital signs will lead to their proper investigation and diagnosis.

Hodgkin's disease (lymphadenoma)

This is a form of lymph node cancer which is characterised by progressive, painless enlargement of lymphoid tissue throughout the body, and anaemia is an associated finding (usually normochromic, normocytic anaemia).

Symptoms include progressive fatigue, loss of weight, large and painless lymph nodes, a large palpable spleen, fever and occasional pruritis. Both sexes are affected, chiefly in adolescence and early adulthood.

Diagnosis is usually established by a lymph node biopsy. Treatment with modern alkylating agents like chlorambucil (Leukeran) can be remarkably successful.

Chronic ciguatera poisoning

Ciguatera is a potent fish-borne toxin that is heat-stable and tasteless. It is concentrated in certain 'gourmet' fish (such as coral trout and some forms of mackerel).

Acute ciguatera poisoning produces neurological, gastro-intestinal and cardiovascular symptoms. A rash and itch are common, together with hypotension (low blood pressure) and bradycardia (slow pulse rate). It is believed that these are produced by the toxin's effect on neuromuscular cell membranes, with a possible autoimmune involvement.

Symptoms usually resolve within weeks, but about 20 per cent of patients remain unwell for months, and less than 2 per cent continue to suffer for years. This latter group usually present with CFS-type symptoms, and are often unaware of the link with ciguatera poisoning.

Those with chronic ciguatera poisoning complain of fatigue, poor exercise tolerance, arthralgia and myalgia. The management is similar to that of CFS, although researchers believe that some cases of chronic ciguatera poisoning are not being identified (with a history of a prior acute attack) and are being labelled as CFS.

Alcoholism

The widespread effects of alcohol abuse can include many of the brain symptoms of CFS (e.g. poor memory, headaches). But liver damage is one of the most common toxic effects, and raised levels of liver enzymes can be confirmed by a simple blood test.

It should be noted that CFS patients have a lower tolerance for alcohol, and a surprisingly small amount can have exaggerated effects. Hypersensitivity to alcohol will be discussed further in Chapter 5.

Hypercalcaemia

This metabolic disorder produces muscle weakness, anorexia, nausea, constipation and excessive thirst. Symptoms have an insidious onset, and, if suspected, diagnosis can be confirmed by a blood calcium level determination.

'Sick building' syndrome

In recent times people have become more aware of the environments in which they live and work. Air-conditioning systems that recycle air, pollutants in our cities and even building materials can affect our immune systems. Headaches, fatigue and a host of other symptoms may occur. The clue to this problem can be the fact that the patient improves dramatically on holiday or at weekends.

More attention to clean, fresh air and the avoidance of potential irritants and allergens are worthwhile. People with respiratory problems (e.g. asthma) and hypersensitivity to house dust mite (causing allergic rhinitis or hay fever) may improve dramatically if carpets are removed, floorboards polished, and soft furnishings are specifically selected to avoid feathers and down. Hydroponic heating and the newer types of vacuum cleaners that feature HEPA filters (high efficiency particulate air filtration) all help to reduce airborne irritants, allergens and infectious agents.

Neoplasm/Tumour

Fatigue itself is non-specific, and several of the symptoms of brain malfunction that occur in CFS could quite easily be the first presenting symptoms of a cerebral tumour. Headaches, balance problems and visual disturbances in particular can be due to the increased intracranial pressure. Brain tissue can be displaced, venous drainage can be obstructed (causing cerebral oedema or swelling), and cerebrospinal fluid circulation impaired.

The symptoms will vary depending on the location of the tumour. A swelling in one cerebral hemisphere may displace the brainstem, and pressure effects are more common if the growth is deep in the hemisphere and especially in the posterior fossa of the brain (described as infratentorial).

Tumours can be benign or malignant. They may be encapsulated and non-infiltrating or, alternately, very rapidly invasive. Symptoms likewise may be due to local pressure only, or they may be caused by a progressively destructive (possibly metastatic) lesion.

It is essential that a brain tumour or lesion be excluded. Early diagnosis and identification of the growth is vital. The problem may be due to other space-occupying lesions such as an abscess or subdural haetoma (collection of blood).

A thorough neurological examination may often reveal signs of a space-occupying lesion causing raised intracranial pressure. The appearance of papilloedema (swelling of the optic disc) and other localising signs (e.g. abnormal reflexes) are important indications of cerebral pathology. Brain scanning is essential, and other investigations including X-rays and angiography may be indicated.

Depending on their accessibility, benign tumours may be completely removed. Even malignant growths, if recognised early, may respond favourably to surgery, radiotherapy or cytotoxic drugs.

Conclusion

It can be seen from the above categories that the causes of fatigue are numerous. Certainly a thorough history must be taken, noting all the symptoms. The combination of symptoms may point towards the likelihood of a diagnosis. And the physical examination must be equally careful in excluding other diagnoses along the way.

Investigations should be chosen that will help rule out any relevant and potentially curable disease that presents with fatigue (as discussed above) and that cannot be excluded by history and examination alone (see suggestions below). Certain blood tests *must* be done, and others should be considered if a real possibility exists of an alternative diagnosis.

Blood tests

There is a growing amount of evidence to suggest chronic, low-level activation of the immune system in CFS, as was discussed in Chapter 2. Recent tests in the USA on a large number of CFS patients were compared with healthy control groups.

Abnormalities in seven tests were found to occur significantly more frequently in CFS patients than in the others. They were: elevated immune complexes, elevated immunoglobulin G, elevated antinuclear antibody titre, elevated alkaline phosphatase, elevated cholesterol, elevated lactic dehydrogenase, and elevated atypical lymphocyte count.

Some of these tests are included on the following list. Others could be added, as each of these tests may support a clinical diagnosis of CFS. However, each test also lacks sufficient sensitivity and specificity to be considered a diagnostic test in its own right. Another complicating factor is the stage of the illness at which the blood is taken. Until there is some standardisation or classification there will always remain room for misinterpretation of results. It is important that patients discuss the place of blood tests (and other investigations) with their doctors.

- Full blood examination (FBE) will reveal:
  - red cell film, including shape, size and number of red cells
  - differential white cell count, indicating the number and proportion of different types of white cells (e.g. lymphocytes, neutophils and eosinophils). It does not give a T-lymphocyte analysis, which is a more complex test used to evaluate immune function. However, this would be relevant if HIV infection were a possibility.
  - platelet count.
- *Erythrocyte sedimentation rate (ESR):* This is a non-specific test that may be elevated in infections, connective tissue disorders and malignancies.
- *Rheumatoid screen:* This includes rheumatoid factor and antinuclear antibody titre; essential to exclude rheumatoid disease.
- *Creatinine kinase:* An enzyme released during muscle damage or pathology; not always raised in CFS patients.
- *Thyroid function tests:* Essential to exclude hypo- or hyperthyroidism.
- *Renal function tests:* Includes urea and electrolytes; serum potassium may be elevated in Addison's disease.
- *Liver functions tests:* These are abnormal in hepatitis, alcoholism and metastatic cancer; they include alkaline phosphatase.
- *Infectious mononucleosis test:* Positive in glandular fever, but not in the early stages.
- *Lyme disease antibodies:* May be appropriate.
- *HIV antibody test:* Important if patient has been at risk.
- *Blood lactic acid:* Frequently elevated in CFS patients after exertion.
- *Blood cortisol:* Reduced in many cases of CFS and severely deficient in Addison's disease.

- *Glutathione level:* An anti-oxidant detoxification substance which is anti-microbial and anti-viral. It is frequently deficient in CFS patients according to Professor Paul Cheney (Director of the Cheney Clinic, USA), who discussed the role of glutathione at the Fatigue 2000 Conference held in the UK in April 1999.

Urinanalysis

Bringing a specimen of urine to your doctor is always worthwhile—not only in fatigue investigation, but also whenever you have a medical check-up. A fresh specimen in a clean screw-top jar will help exclude many conditions. By simply dipping a laboratory strip into the specimen your doctor can immediately establish the presence or absence of blood, protein, glucose, ketones, liver breakdown products and other substances. This simple screening test can be done on the spot by the GP. And should a more detailed examination or culture (to look for possible infection) be necessary, your doctor will ask you to provide a further specimen— collected mid-stream into a sterile container.

Researchers from the University of Newcastle in Australia have reported altered metabolite excretion in the urine of CFS patients. The discovery of anomalies in the excretion of certain amino acids and organic acids (CFSUMI and beta-alanine) implicate these metabolites in the pathophysiology of CFS, in particular by their effects on neurotransmission and energy utilisation. These findings suggest that a definite object-diagnostic test for CFS may possibly eventuate.

Radiology

A current chest X-ray may well be indicated if you have been feverish or coughing, or have a past history of smoking or possible contact with tuberculosis.

Specific joint X-rays are required where there has been a localised arthralgia (joint pain). They may also be necessary in cases of possible referred pain. Headaches could be due to referred pain from a degenerative disc in the neck. A film of the cervical spine will show if this is the case.

Scanning

A brain scan is very important when investigating the cerebral symptoms of CFS. One cannot assume that symptoms of brain malfunction (as discussed in Chapter 2) are due to CFS or any other condition where the possibility of a cerebral tumour or other space-occupying lesion has not been ruled out.

Magnetic resonance imaging (MRI) will also show the characteristic lesions of multiple sclerosis, which is an important differential diagnosis.

Summary

The investigations involve a number of blood tests, urin-analysis, X-rays and scanning. No two patients are identical, although there are many symptoms in common. The final choice of tests will be made by your doctor, who will have first taken a thorough history and then performed a physical examination. The results of the investigations will then enable an accurate diagnosis to be made.

Chapter five

Treatment of CFS

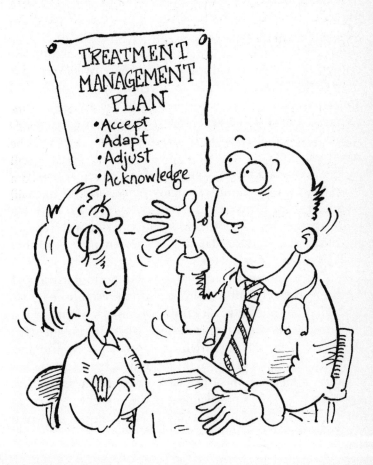

Once CFS has been diagnosed an overall plan of management must be drawn up. There are many issues to be addressed as the illness affects every aspect of a patient's life. Every situation is unique and the presenting problems will vary from patient to patient, although disabling fatigue is common to all.

A majority of patients will feel some relief at their illness being identified. Although the chronicity and limitations imposed by CFS are nothing to celebrate, the fear of having a terminal illness is much worse. When one has never been ill and is suddenly stopped in one's tracks it is only natural to think of all the possibilities. Like so many other things in life we tend to take good health for granted until it is compromised in some way.

For the vast majority of CFS sufferers there is reason for optimism. All the studies and research have shown that most CFS patients *do get better*—eventually! The outlook is at least hopeful, even if the length of the illness cannot be predicted. What does seem to improve the prognosis is the correct management of the illness from the time it is identified.

The duration of symptoms in a CFS patient can range from just over six months to many years, with the average length of illness between three to five years. As we learn more about CFS it becomes more apparent that the earlier the diagnosis, the more favourable the outcome. And that will depend on your doctor.

It is an unfortunate fact that many important aspects of medicine are still to find their way into the established texts and syllabi of our university training schools. Medicine is a notoriously conservative profession where, although standards are high, the unknown or unproven is regarded as dubious. Perhaps it is fear of the unknown; but in the case of CFS it is a fact that must be faced. Over recent years there has been a marked improvement in the amount of research into CFS, especially in the United Kingdom, the USA and Australia. Those dedicated research teams have steadily built up a large bank of knowledge that is at last being given due recognition. There is still much to learn, but at least there are doctors in our society who do take CFS seriously, as it deserves to be.

In the previous chapter I stated that most doctors now accept CFS as a real illness. Unfortunately many, through ignorance or prejudice, see it as a 'waste-basket' diagnosis and fail to follow through. They have little idea of the correct management and feel inadequate in treating a complex disorder for which there is no easy cure. Some are genuinely concerned about labelling a patient's condition as CFS because of the possible impact it may have upon the patient!

A minority of doctors even fail to acknowledge the existence of CFS. They feel threatened by a set of symptoms for which they have no ready explanation. It is often so much easier to label a patient a 'hypochondriac' or their symptoms as 'psychosomatic'. To make matters worse, some patients, in their anxiety, have already been to several doctors and have gained an unfair reputation for 'doctor shopping'.

Mrs P was one such patient. She came to me in desperation at the very time I was reducing my workload. A highly intelligent woman, she had developed a fairly typical history of fatigue, myalgia and sleep disturbance, superimposed on menopausal symptoms for which she took hormone replacement therapy. Her brother was a longstanding patient of mine who was very concerned when his sister had been sent to a psychiatrist and admitted to a local hospital. The psychiatrist, after assessing her further, had discharged her without finding any psychiatric cause for her symptoms. Understandably she was unwilling to continue with her former GP. In due course she was confirmed as having CFS, and has since made great progress with a physician of my choice.

A more tragic tale was brought to my attention at a recent seminar. This particular case involved a seventeen-year-old boy who was having difficulties at school. He had apparently never recovered fully from a viral infection and progressed to what, in hindsight, was a classic case of CFS. His illness was never properly investigated and his condition deteriorated. It was commonly thought he was suffering 'stress', until his suicide shocked some of the local rural community into re-evaluating his situation. They later realised that his symptoms had been trivialised and he felt isolated from family, friends and a particularly dismissive GP.

The advantages of a definite diagnosis are clear. The sooner a patient is properly evaluated the better. Few people are pleased to know they have a chronic condition. However, they will almost invariably prefer a diagnosis which explains their debilitating condition and gives meaning to their months, or years, of suffering. Studies are now emerging which confirm that lack of an early diagnosis in CFS is related to deteriorating health and a poor prognosis.

Any illness for which there is no specific treatment will attract the attention of alternative 'practitioners'. It is hardly surprising that alternative approaches have attracted a following, especially since many GPs feel uneasy about dealing with an illness for which they do not have all the answers. My advice here is to take care!

In this chapter we will examine many forms of treatment, some 'conventional' and some 'alternative'. I have no intention of casting aspersions on the latter but I do urge CFS patients to tread carefully. Many of these practitioners mean well, but the claims made by some hardly give them credibility.

It is a misapprehension that all 'natural' medicines are harmless. The fact that a substance may be naturally occurring or 'just another vitamin or trace element' does not necessarily make it safe—especially in the mega-doses advised by some. And many of these therapies are not available on the subsidised health schemes, making them expensive as well.

Another problem with some alternative treatments is the great hope invested in them. While there is nothing wrong in having faith in a particular treatment, it is an unfortunate fact that some CFS patients may be grasping at straws. Weakened by their debilitating illness, they build up an unrealistic expectation. If there is no improvement, they emerge from the experiment with shattered hopes and feeling worse than ever.

It is my sincere belief that a CFS patient, once diagnosed, should remain under medical care. If the patient's own doctor is not confident dealing with CFS, then it is imperative that the patient be referred to a doctor who is. The role of the doctor is to coordinate management, give supportive advice, prescribe any necessary medication, and consider all treatment options frankly with the patient. If the patient is tempted by some alternative treatment, then this can be discussed. There are many cases where successful treatment has been an intelligent blend of conventional medicine with alternative therapy. But it is important for that balance to exist.

Treating the symptoms

The most prominent symptoms to be treated in CFS are:
- fatigue
- muscle pain
- mood changes
- headaches
- sleep disturbances.

The many other symptoms, as discussed in Chapter 3, are less constant. They form a variable clinical picture and require treatment when, and if, they arise.

Fatigue is the most persistent debilitating symptom of all. It is the most limiting and restrictive aspect of the illness, especially for a patient who has always been active and well. And it is the fatigue that dictates the mainstay of treatment. If the fatigue is ignored, then the other symptoms follow in quick pursuit. One of the most difficult aspects of treating CFS is learning to recognise when the fatigue is starting to occur. Unlike a normal fit person, the CFS patient cannot ignore the warnings. To do so is to invite a relapse that may take days of total rest to get over.

At the first sign of tired muscles it is essential to stop the activity. If you push beyond this early point to the stage of fatigue, then it will take hours to recover from the muscle pain and feelings of abnormal fatigue. Should you ignore both these points (tiredness, fatigue) and continue exercising to the point of exhaustion, then the recovery phase will be measured in days instead of hours. The golden rule is 'When walking or doing any physical activity, obey the first feelings of **tiredness**. Do not push yourself to the **fatigue** stage, and never to the stage of **exhaustion**.'

What is interpreted by a normal person as 'a healthy tiredness' is an ominous sign for a CFS patient. In the early stages of the illness even trivial exertion will cause fatigue, and put that person totally out of action for hours or days. Rest is an absolute necessity and, quite logically, heads the list of treatments.

In all CFS patients the treatment is made up of the following:
- Rest
- Medications
- Modified exercise
- Diet
- Alternative therapies
- Spinal decompression surgery (in selected cases).

Rest

In the early stages of CFS this usually means bed rest for most patients. But, as every case is different, it is ultimately the severity of the symptoms that dictates the degree of immobilisation. It is only when lying down that the muscles are totally relaxed, and exhaustion is followed by a return to a restful state. It is at this time that you feel at your weakest and most vulnerable. The bed becomes your 'safe haven' and, despite the restrictions, offers the only option.

Many patients have vivid recollections of their CFS at its most severe and limiting. My own experience was of spending several weeks in bed, interrupted only by several hours a day sitting out of bed or being driven to the doctor or some similar outing. Social contact was mostly by phone and my feelings of isolation were relieved by those wonderful patients and friends who rang at regular intervals to make sure I was 'still in the land of the living'.

Feeling helpless and despondent is a fact of life for CFS sufferers. You must accept that you cannot do the things you would normally take for granted. The small amount of energy available is used up on doing the most basic tasks. Having a bath or shower and sitting up for a meal would be followed by several hours of total rest to restore one's minimal energy balance.

Your bed almost becomes the centre of your existence. During these weeks or months you realise that life must and will go on without you. All your effort and energy are used for the most basic of lifestyles. A trip to the bathroom or kitchen becomes an excursion, and to go outside to the letterbox is almost an adventure!

The dangers of prolonged bed rest are well known. It is rather unsettling to know you are not using your muscles or joints properly, and that they may suffer from disuse. However, muscle wasting is not common in CFS and, in any case, it is hardly a consideration when one is in pain. And the joints will still move when you have enough energy to exercise them. It seems that our bodies know best most of the time.

Medications

All medications should be taken for good reason. It is important to avoid the problems of drug interactions or the potentiation of one drug's action by the taking of another. With CFS, it will be necessary at times to be on several medications at the same time, so they should be taken (and prescribed) with care.

It is important to discuss any addition to your medications with your doctor before starting these. Even vitamin supplements should be discussed as these may be toxic in some patients; especially bearing in mind that as part of their condition CFS patients tend to be hypersensitive to drugs. To complicate matters some of the drugs most commonly prescribed in CFS may have side-effects, which may in fact exacerbate the symptoms. So, on the one hand, their effect may be beneficial, while, on the other, they may have an undesirable action.

The drugs most commonly used in CFS are:

- anti-inflammatory drugs (non steroidal)
- analgesics
- antidepressants
- antibiotics.

Non-steroidal anti-inflammatory drugs

As discussed in Chapter 3, anti-inflammatory drugs are useful to control muscle pain in most situations. A small regular dose given once or twice daily (after a meal) may be necessary to keep myalgia to a minimum. But some patients find they only need to use them sporadically, especially in the later stages of the illness.

There are many drugs within this group. They include indomethacin (Indocid), ketoprofen (Orudis), naproxen (Naprosyn), piroxicam (Feldene), sulindac (Clinoril), as well as aspirin. Most have been available for years, and some are specially formulated to be released slowly after ingestion ('S-R' means sustained release), thus ensuring a constant level in the blood over a longer period.

This group of drugs can have a major adverse effect on the gastrointestinal system. They may cause abdominal pain, nausea, drowsiness, headaches, dizziness, skin rashes and, in some, visual disturbances and raised liver enzymes in the blood. But their major drawback is their propensity to cause gastric ulceration and gastrointestinal bleeding.

Quite obviously, any patient with a history of peptic ulceration or a tendency to bleed should not take this group of anti-inflammatory drugs. And in those who can tolerate them, they must never be taken on an empty stomach.

Over the years the problems with oral anti-inflammatory drugs have led to some improvements in their administration. Several of these medications are available in suppository form and work very well when inserted rectally. A few are available as a spray or a gel that can be applied topically to those muscles involved. This is a great advantage if there is localised muscle or joint involvement. However, CFS tends to be more generalised in its effect and oral or rectal administration is preferable in most situations.

Anti-inflammatory drugs should only be taken with your doctor's approval and should not be given to children under twelve years of age. Any possible side-effects must be reported and the medication either modified, changed or stopped. Used carefully they are excellent drugs which give great relief in the muscle pain of CFS. Their other major long-term use is in the treatment of arthritis (both rheumatoid and osteo-) and fibromyalgia syndrome, which was discussed in Chapter 4.

A more controversial area is the use of steroidal agents in CFS. Corticosteroids have occasionally been used when there has been no marked improvement with the nonsteroidal anti-inflammatory drugs. However, the potential for side-effects and the need for careful monitoring make this a much riskier treatment, which must be carefully supervised by your doctor.

Anabolic steroids are not available for general use in Australia. They have received much publicity for their (illicit) use in enhancing the performance of sports personalities in various fields. They may seem especially attractive to some CFS sufferers. But, again, their use must be strictly monitored, and the risk of long-term toxic effects must be taken into consideration.

Analgesics

With the exception of aspirin, analgesics have very little anti-inflammatory action. They are used primarily for pain that has not responded to anti-inflammatory medication or where the use of anti-inflammatory drugs is contra-indicated.

Paracetamol (under various brand names) is readily available over the counter and is probably the most widely used analgesic. It also has the advantage of being safe to use in children. With any medication, however, there is a maximum dosage and, in adults, this is eight tablets of 500 g over a 24-hour period (usually taken as two tablets six-hourly). Even this amount should not be taken for a prolonged period. Adverse effects include dyspepsia, nausea, skin rashes and haematological changes, which are evident on a full blood examination. Prolonged use can also cause impairment to kidney and liver function. If the pain is not being adequately controlled, then you must look at a stronger analgesic such as codeine.

Codeine can be taken on its own or combined with aspirin or paracetamol for greater effect. It is ideal for moderate pain relief where paracetamol is found to be insufficient; or it may be used in addition to an anti-inflammatory drug for those times when, during a relapse of CFS, the muscle pain is persistent. Higher doses of codeine are constipating, and other side-effects include nausea, dizziness and sedation.

Stronger analgesia should not be necessary in CFS if the muscles are rested, warmth applied, and the patient remains in bed during a relapse. Most patients will respond to codeine. However, in those patients who suffer a severe headache there may occasionally be a case for stronger analgesic drugs. But these are only available on prescription, and the risk of dependency must be considered by both patient and doctor.

Antidepressants

The role of antidepressants in the treatment of CFS has already been mentioned. Understandably, depression is a common consequence of any chronic illness. But the extent to which a patient is affected has a great deal to do with his or her personality before the illness, and the extent to which the patient can cope with the limitations imposed by the illness.

Before CFS attracted such attention from medical researchers there was (and unfortunately still is) a lack of understanding by some sections of the medical profession. When confronted by the diverse symptomatology of CFS, the GP would tend to focus on the brain-related symptoms of sleep disturbances and mood change. The problem would be considered primarily a psychiatric one. In desperation, some GPs referred their CFS patients to a psychiatrist, but in many cases they were sent back without a primary psychiatric disorder being diagnosed.

The role of antidepressants in CFS is an interesting one. For some years it was thought that patients with a significant depression would benefit from this group of drugs. Many trials later it became apparent that in some instances the patient's mood was indeed improved, but the antidepressants had no effect whatsoever on the primary problem of fatigue.

One Dutch study went so far as to say that, in a double-blind trial, fluoxetine (Prozac) appeared to have no effect on depression, fatigue or any other feature associated with CFS. This suggests that a totally different process was at work in CFS patients, as opposed to those with a major depressive disorder where the benefits of this drug are well known.

There are several other important reasons why this appears to be so. First, there is a group of symptoms in CFS that does not reflect psychiatric illness. These symptoms include the syndrome's sudden onset, lymph-node enlargement and post-exertional malaise. Second, studies have shown abnormalities of the brain in the hypothalamic-pituitary axis that are quite different to what one sees in major depression or other psychiatric illness. Third, there is the failure of CFS to resolve fully with psychiatric therapy, including antidepressant drugs.

I discussed hypothalamic-pituitary dysfunction in Chapter 2. In brief, the hypothalamus makes hormones that affect the pituitary gland. And the pituitary gland makes hormones that affect the adrenal glands. In healthy people a normal amount is made by each of these glands. In major depression a very high amount of these chemicals is made by each organ. But in CFS the situation is the exact opposite—an underproduction by the pituitary of adreno-corticotrophic hormone, which leads to an underproduction of cortisol by the adrenal glands. This objective measure in CFS is different from the normal population and even more so from patients suffering major depression.

It appears that some antidepressants do help the depression that often occurs as a result of CFS, without having any effect on the other symptoms or on the actual course of the illness itself. It is for this reason that the use of an anti-depressant is often indicated, and justifiably so. I discussed the symptoms of depression in Chapter 4 and before look-ing at the various types available, it is worth noting that not all cases of depression require drugs. In fact, in the milder cases of depression a patient can benefit greatly from certain 'self-help measures', which may be all that is necessary to change one's mood.

In any chronic illness, depression may be a complicating factor. The chances of this occurring are lessened consider-ably if the patient thinks positively and keeps mentally active. No matter how bad you may feel physically, there are many ways to lift the mood. Feelings of anger and frus-tration, although understandable, are negative and often destructive. It is worthwhile to keep the mind actively involved with new interests and ongoing commitments.

Books, music, radio and television are all therapeutic if used selectively and wisely.

Talking and keeping in touch with friends are also therapeutic. For the bed-bound, the telephone is a great aid. When able, do try to get out to a few social events, even if you have to sit down for most of the time. It is not a good idea to cut off all social contact. And remember, your doctor is there to share your concerns and lighten the load. Referral to a psychiatrist is also an option if you are having difficulty coping, but is unnecessary in most cases.

If an antidepressant is thought necessary, there is a wide variety from which to choose. The three main groups are:

- tricyclics
- monoamine oxidase inhibitors
- 5-hydroxytryptamine (5 HT) re-uptake inhibitors.

i *Tricyclics:* This group remains the most widely prescribed and, it appears, the most suitable for treating depression in CFS. They take several weeks before having an obvious effect, so it is important to give them time to reach their therapeutic level. Dosage also needs to be individualised for best results.

One of the drawbacks is possible side-effects. All tricyclics can cause dry mouth, constipation, weight gain, dizziness and a fall in blood pressure. However, these tend to be a problem only with higher dosages and can be avoided by commencing the patient on a low dosage and gradually building up over a period of several weeks. Giving the entire dose at night tends to lessen the problems and may even be therapeutic in those patients made drowsy by such medication. However, this group's symptoms of fatigue could be worsened by this sedating effect.

Tricyclics should be used with extra care in some patients. Anyone with a history of cardiovascular disorders, hyperthyroidism, diabetes or glaucoma needs regular supervision. And in elderly males with urinary retention problems (from enlarged prostate glands) this treatment may not be suitable. Women who are pregnant or breastfeeding should also have their dosage closely monitored.

Adverse interactions may also be a problem with tricyclic antidepressants. Alcohol can exacerbate their effect, while other antidepressants, anticholinergics and sympathomimetic drugs have undesirable effects and should be avoided. Patients on MAO-inhibitor drugs (see below) or those who have suffered a recent heart attack (myocardial infarct) should never be given tricyclic antidepressants.

ii *Monoamine oxidase (MAO) inhibitors:* This group acts by inhibiting the action of a specific enzyme in the brain (MAO). They tend to be used in situations where depression is atypical or where there are associated problems such as phobic anxiety. They are also used where the tricyclics are less effective, and some doctors consider them superior in treating those cases of depression where lethargy is prominent.

Indeed, studies at Sydney's Prince Henry Hospital where the drug 'moclobemide' (Aurorix), a reversible MAO inhibitor, was compared with a placebo showed that this antidepressant was especially effective in CFS patients who had impaired cell-mediated immunity (indicated by reduced T-cell levels). The results suggested moclobemide may improve patients' fatigue, whether or not depression was significant. The lack of side-effects (especially sedation) was seen as a great advantage.

The main drawback with MAO inhibitor drugs is their interaction with tyramine, a chemical found in many foods and other drugs (beer, cheese, Bovril, Oxo, certain decongestant mixtures). This can provoke a hypertensive crisis, with splitting headache and a risk of sub-arachnoid haemorrhage. MAO inhibitors also potentiate the effect of many other drugs including opiates, phenothiazines and alcohol.

iii *5-hydroxytryptamine (5 HT) re-uptake inhibitors:* This more recent group of antidepressants (e.g. fluoxetine) acts by increasing the levels of a chemical called 5-hydroxytrypt-amine (5 HT) in the brain. These drugs have significantly fewer side-effects than the tricyclics but can cause nausea, anorexia, sweating and tremors. But all these side-effects tend to diminish after the first few weeks of treatment. They must not be used for at least several weeks after a course of MAO inhibitors; and, in reverse, MAO inhibitors must not be used for at least five weeks after stopping them. They may also interact with other antidepressants and phenothiazines.

Interestingly, fluoxetine has been shown to be of little or no benefit to CFS patients in a recent Dutch trial. The placebo-controlled double-blind study showed that even in doses up to four times the normal therapeutic dose for depression, there was no real improvement for the CFS patient, either in their fatigue or their depression.

It has become apparent that some CFS patients, with or without depressive symptoms, may benefit from a tailored dose of either moclobemide (a reversible MAO inhibitor) or one of the tricyclic drugs. Any depressive symptoms resulting from CFS should improve. And, perhaps even more importantly, the ability to cope with the overwhelming muscular fatigue may be enhanced, allowing one to get on with life.

Antibiotics

Antibiotics appear to be of little use in CFS. If there is a trigger factor known to respond (e.g. Lyme disease), then of course treatment is indicated. Likewise, a concurrent bacterial infection must have the appropriate antibiotic, as any untreated infection will certainly cause a relapse in the symptoms of CFS. However, the prescription of an antibiotic must be justified, and it must be taken for its full course unless there is some reason (e.g. allergic reaction) to stop it and change to a different one.

There has been much publicity about the overprescription of antibiotics in recent years. With the emergence of increasingly resistant strains of bacteria this presents a frightening scenario. It is no exaggeration to say that, within a few years, we could see great epidemics occurring as in ages past. The armament of antibacterial drugs we have is looking less effective by the year, and even the development of new drugs is not keeping pace with the bacterial mutations and threat of untreatable infections.

There was a theory that CFS may be helped by tetracycline therapy. I am unsure how it originated but I can find no evidence to justify the long-term use of any antibacterial drug in the treatment of CFS.

Modified exercise

One of the most difficult aspects of managing CFS is knowing how much one needs to exercise. In the early stages of the illness exercising at all is often out of the question. When the most trivial physical pursuits can precipitate hours or even days of muscle pain and exhaustion, then the very thought of an exercise routine becomes ludicrous.

However, the dangers of remaining bound to a bed or a chair are equally worrying. Muscles and joints need to move, and our knowledge of heart disease decrees that we should all try to adhere to a healthy exercise program. The best solution appears to be a compromise.

During this time of enforced bed rest it is wise at least to move the muscles in bed. Flexing and extending the ankle, knee and hip joints need not bring on pain if performed slowly and in moderation. The lower limb muscles tend to be the most neglected when immobilised, so a program of gentle mobilisation is advisable.

Baths are preferable to showers. Not only are they more relaxing; they offer the chance for daily hydrotherapy. I found (and still find) that a warm bath on first rising is good inducement for the joints to go through their paces. Again, a sensible number of flexion-extension exercises (start with five) and some gentle rotation of hips and shoulder joints will improve your mobility and exercise muscles that have otherwise been ignored.

Walking on flat ground around the house or in the garden or street is a good routine to establish. Even if most of your time is necessarily spent in bed there should be several times a day when you can get up and walk a little. With the progression of time a patient becomes better able to judge when muscles are becoming sore and fatigue is imminent. By heeding these signs and returning to bed you will at least have had some gentle exercise between the periods of bed rest. And, most importantly, you will not have gone beyond the point of fatigue—let alone the point of exhaustion.

As the weeks turn to months, the amount of walking can usually be increased. But you will still have days when you are unable to do almost any exercise. These 'bad' days will eventually become less frequent and less severe, but they will still persist in many patients for several years.

The restriction on one's social life is obvious. It is advisable to try to get out for a few hours several times a week. This may necessitate having flexible arrangements, but it is better than none at all. For psychological reasons, if no other, it is important to have some social contact as the acute phase of the illness subsides. Attending a small dinner party or enjoying a night at the movies or theatre is a welcome break from the bedroom, even if dressing for the occasion uses your entire energy allowance for the day!

As CFS progresses from the acute phase it is advisable to incorporate a small amount of aerobic exercise into the daily routine. I have already mentioned the benefits of walking. Other pursuits may include swimming or even jogging on a rebounder. But the limits to which a patient can go are restrictive. It is far better to achieve a modest goal rather than end up in bed the entire next day for being too ambitious.

Walking on flat ground or swimming in a warm pool is the safest way of keeping fit. You are more likely to be able to pace yourself and sustain a mild to moderate level of activity without reaching the danger zones of tiredness, fatigue or exhaustion. If you stop at the first feeling of tiredness you will be able to get a good idea of your capability and limits for future sessions. Remember the golden rule mentioned earlier: 'When walking or doing any physical activity, obey the first feelings of **tiredness**. Do not push yourself to the **fatigue** stage and never to the stage of **exhaustion**.'

The benefits of a graded aerobic exercise program have recently been shown to be of enormous value in CFS patients. In fact, for the general public as well, this is an excellent way to keep fit. Apart from the obvious positive effects on the cardiovascular system, a sustainable exercise program will improve immune function, reduce stress and protect muscles and joints from prolonged periods of inactivity. And in the majority of patients at one London CFS clinic, symptoms were noticeably improved after a year of graded supervised aerobic exercise treatments.

Another very important reason to exercise is weight control. It is quite apparent that decreased physical activity will burn up fewer calories, tip the scales in an unfavourable direction and increase the waistline. Even with a sensible diet (see below) it is very easy to take in more calories or kilojoules than we are actually using up. And there is quite enough to get depressed about with CFS without having to cope with being overweight as well!

Diet

There are few areas of general practice more important than preventive medicine. And, in that department, lifestyle and dietary principles top the list. So many illnesses are either caused or worsened by a poor diet. Living in a fast-moving, westernised society (which we sometimes mistakenly label as 'sophisticated') may actually aggravate the problem.

So much has been written about diet and nutrition that I feel almost apologetic in adding to the literature. And yet it never ceases to amaze me how much space is taken up in the magazines and popular press by the latest fad or 'miracle' diet that promises model-like figures, glowing health and abundant energy. It all appears so complicated. But it need not, believe me!

No diet or food alone can guarantee good health. Health depends on many factors, including heredity, lifestyle, attitudes and environment. But the following dietary guidelines will:

- maximise energy levels in CFS
- control weight
- lower blood cholesterol and cardiovascular disease
- reduce the risk of cancers
- help prevent diabetes
- protect against diverticular disease and other bowel problems.

To have one dietary plan that accomplishes *all* of these is much simpler than measuring calories or eliminating certain foods altogether and risking the dangers of an unbalanced diet. Good nutrition can be fun. Learning a few simple principles is easy and of inestimable value, whether you have a chronic illness or just want to remain healthy.

Certainly, calories or kilojoules are important. If you take in 2500 calories a day and burn up only 2000, then you will gradually put on weight. But if you follow my suggested dietary plan the calories will look after themselves.

You will notice that nothing is completely forbidden on my suggested diet. It simply advises to increase certain food types and decrease others. Apart from decreasing the incidence of all the severe medical disorders listed above, the majority of my patients who followed these dietary principles found that they retained their ideal weight, or lost weight if they needed to. Apart from it being the healthiest, most liberal diet most of my patients had ever been advised, they almost unanimously reported feeling better. And their body weights in most cases achieved an equilibrium. So much so that, in twenty years of practice, I seldom had to prescribe an appetite suppressant.

There are three main terms that must be remembered—all food should be judged bearing them in mind. They are:

- **fats** (especially saturated fats)
- **sugars** (or refined carbohydrates), and
- **alcohol**.

I advocate a diet that is high in protein, complex carbohydrates, vitamins and fibre, and low in fats, sugar and alcohol. I emphasised the last three terms as I find it is often easier to look at food and assess its nutritional value first from a negative point of view. If it is low in fats, sugars and alcohol, then there is a good chance it will be healthy.

We derive energy from our food. The average westernised diet contains about 40 per cent of calories or kilojoules as fat, 15 per cent as protein and 45 per cent as carbohydrates. To achieve a healthier nutrition we should reduce fat content to 25 per cent, increase protein to about 20 per cent and increase carbohydrates to about 55 per cent.

Fats

The type of fat in our diet is important. Fats can be derived from animals or plants, and may be polyunsaturated, monounsaturated or saturated, referring to the fatty acids that make them up. Many dietary fats are a mixture of all three, but it is important to differentiate between them.

Saturated fats are usually solid, of animal origin and found in dairy produce and in meats. But some vegetable oils are also saturated (coconut and palm oils) and used in the production of pastries and biscuits. Foods high in saturates increase the blood cholesterol level.

Polyunsaturated fats are usually liquid and of plant origin (safflower, sunflower, maize), but can also be found in some fish oils (omega-3 type) where they reduce the blood's tendency to clot. The polyunsaturated group can actually help to lower blood cholesterol levels.

Monounsaturated fats are found in both animals and plants. Olive oil is more than 75 per cent monounsaturated. Whereas saturated fats tend to raise cholesterol and polyunsaturated fats tend to lower it, monounsaturated fats have an intermediate effect, but are beneficial in the absence of saturates.

Cholesterol is always animal derived and found in brain, liver, kidney, egg yolk and prawns. Contrary to popular belief, it is not so much these foods that influence blood cholesterol as the amount of saturated fats in the diet.

In brief, you should aim to include only polyunsaturates and monounsaturates in the diet. However, all are equally caloric and even the 'good' fats should only be eaten sparingly if weight is a problem.

Carbohydrates

Carbohydrates should mostly be of the complex kind. Cereals, grains and breads are examples that also contain a high amount of dietary fibre. This fibre is not absorbed and helps to clear cholesterol products from the digestive system.

Breads should be wholemeal, rye or the soy-and-linseed combination. In addition to being high in fibre, the latter provides alpha-linolenic acid, which is converted to the same beneficial omega-3 polyunsaturated fatty acids found in fish and known to have a beneficial cardiovascular effect. It also provides a significant intake of phytoestrogens (natural compounds similar to the hormone oestrogen). Four slices a day will provide about two-thirds of the recommended daily fibre intake.

The complex carbohydrate foods provide a sustained moderate amount of energy, as opposed to the sudden high peak that occurs when eating sugar (which is a refined rather than complex carbohydrate). Sugar can also raise blood triglyceride levels (a cardiovascular risk factor) as well as predisposing an individual to diabetes.

The sustained moderate levels of energy provided by a diet high in complex carbohydrates are not only more preferable for patients with CFS. They are also advisable in anyone who wishes to avoid the 'highs and lows' in normal blood sugar levels, which can occur throughout the course of a day in someone who is on a more erratic diet.

Alcohol

Alcohol should be kept to a minimum. It provides 'empty calories'—that is, it will put on weight without providing much other nourishment. In excessive amounts it is responsible for many health problems (including liver disease), but, used sparingly, it can be beneficial in reducing the blood's tendency to clot. It therefore has a cardio-protective effect. It is well known that the French have a relatively low incidence of cardiovascular disease despite an abundance of saturated fat in their diet (meat, butter, cream). Their traditional and liberal use of wine is almost certainly the reason; the alcohol tending to neutralise the effect of the fats.

It is not uncommon for CFS patients to have a markedly lower tolerance for alcohol. They may well feel better not taking it at all. And in patients with a weight problem, the benefits of cutting out alcohol (and those 'empty' calories) are very soon apparent. But, used sensibly in conjunction with a healthy diet, there is nothing nicer than a glass or two of a good wine with the evening meal.

I have already mentioned fibre under complex carbohydrates. Other foods high in fibre include fruit and vegetables, which are also important sources of vitamins and minerals. These should be included at every meal. Not only is their nutritional value high, but they are a good substitute for some of the fatty 'snack' foods found in most westernised diets.

High protein foods include meat, chicken and seafood.

These should be trimmed of visible fat (including skin in the case of poultry). This not only reduces the caloric content but cuts down the overall intake of fat. The amount of meat per serve should be 100–150 g (after removing fat, skin and bones). Even apparently lean meats will still contain some fat, but it will be minimised. Asian dishes are especially healthy as they tend to use even less meat and increase the proportion of vegetables and rice.

A diet that rotates red and white meats is ideal. Fish should be included at least twice a week as it is low in fat, yet has a higher proportion of the valuable omega-3 polyunsaturates that are cardio-protective. The preferred modes of cooking for meats, poultry and seafood are grilling, baking, stir-frying or steaming. Poaching fish and cooking meat as casseroles are also recommended, depending on the type of cuisine. Where cooking oil is required it should be either polyunsaturated or monounsaturated (e.g. olive oil).

Vegetarian diets need not differ greatly. But instead of meat, poultry or seafood, you would use a greater variety of lentils, beans, nuts and eggs. Vegetables should be either cooked in a steamer within a saucepan, simmered with a minimal amount of water or baked in the oven. Microwaving is also possible (and very convenient), but again the amount of water used should be minimal. In Asian dishes vegetables can be stir-fried or steamed.

The larger variety of foods required in a vegetarian diet is necessary to provide the protein. Proteins are made up of amino acids, of which about 20 or so are termed 'essential' because we cannot manufacture them ourselves. Full complements are available in meat, poultry and seafoods but vegetarian food sources are always deficient in some of the essential amino acids. This need not be a problem if a sufficiently diverse range of protein foods is included in the vegetarian diet. A healthy vegetarian needs to be aware of this and plan his or her diet accordingly.

A sample menu:

BREAKFAST

Stewed fruit/prunes (preferable to fruit juice)
Weetbix/rolled oats with low-fat milk
Toast (wholemeal/rye/soy-linseed) with a small
amount of polyunsaturated margarine and
marmalade/ honey/ jam

LUNCH

Sandwiches (wholemeal/rye/soy-linseed) containing
skinless chicken/lean beef/ham/smoked salmon
with various salad constituents (lettuce, tomato,
cucumber etc.)
Piece of fruit, peeled or well washed

DINNER

Roast beef/lamb/pork(lean) OR
Grilled steak (lean fillet or rump) OR
Roast chicken without skin OR
Grilled/steamed/baked fish,
served with at least three (preferably four) vegetables,
including a green variety (all
steamed/microwaved/baked)
Alternatively, the main course may consist of a
stir-fried or steamed Asian dish OR
Italian pasta dish OR
Casserole (meat/chicken/fish)
with the vegetables incorporated or served separately
Steamed rice is an ideal alternative to potatoes

DESSERT

Should preferably be fruit-based or a pudding served
with reduced-fat icecream or cream

Alcohol should be restricted to two to three standard drinks for men, or one to two for women. This includes any spirits or beer before dinner as well as red/white wine with dinner.

Tea or coffee can be taken during the day, but not late in the evening unless decaffeinated.

At least eight glasses or cups of fluid should be taken daily, including liberal amounts of water.

This menu is a guide only and is a reflection of the high protein/complex carbohydrate and low fat/sugar/alcohol content of the ideal diet.

The increase in Asian and European-style cuisine over the past few decades has been very beneficial to all Australians. New vegetables, herbs and flavours have made food more interesting, and the variety of ingredients is amazing. Even the humble potato now comes in many different types, and a visit to the market is quite educational. The vast array of seafood available is a pleasing sight, as is the interest taken in cooking by both sexes, young and old.

It adds interest to incorporate some different styles of cuisine into your diet. And many of the best dishes are high in protein, complex carbohydrates and fibre while being low in fats and sugars. They also tend to be low in calories providing the serves are of reasonable size. Once you develop a taste for a diet that is lower in fats, then you will generally prefer to keep it that way. Patients who have cut down the fat content of their milk (for weight or cholesterol reasons) inevitably adjust to it. Re-educating the palate along these lines means that if you sometimes lapse it doesn't really matter. It is what you eat **most** of the time that will determine your overall health.

Fast foods

Despite an increase in public awareness of good nutrition there has been a proliferation of fast-food outlets in recent decades. The very pace of modern living has made the convenience of 'junk food' an attraction for many, especially the younger age groups. And they have been aided and coerced by the advertising agencies.

The image of the health-conscious young family is one that has been carefully fostered by big business. Even the models we see tucking into this type of food are slim, young and attractive—a far cry from the real picture. For most westernised nations are battling with a mortality rate that is needlessly high, with an ever-increasing health bill made worse by hospitals bulging at the seams with patients who are largely responsible for their own ill-health.

The list of preventable illnesses affecting the so-called 'well-off' nations would fill a textbook. Obesity, diabetes, coronary heart disease and cancer are mostly related to lifestyle; and nutrition is about the most important aspect of lifestyle because it is something over which we ourselves have control.

Many other illnesses, including abnormalities of the immune system (e.g. CFS) are aggravated by poor nutrition. It is ironic that, in an age where there have been great advances in nutritional science, the 'junk-food mentality' still rules in many lives. Despite a so-called 'high standard of living' we still see apparently sensible adults poisoning their systems with junk food, often costing as much or more than good-quality food that would take minimal time and effort to prepare in their own home. Today we have the benefits of microwave ovens and freezers, so there is really little excuse.

Fast foods are not necessarily 'junk foods', but tend to be. It is possible to order something nutritious on the run, but that, unfortunately, is the exception. Most fast foods are very high in saturated fats (which will increase blood cholesterol levels), sugar and, of course, calories. Apart from a slim, healthy and vocal minority, today's diets and life-styles are increasingly creating a nation of overweight couch potatoes, with arteries that are clogging up at an ever-increasing rate from an ever-decreasing age. That, sadly, is the truth.

Children are most susceptible to advertising. It takes a great deal of time and effort for parents and schools to re-educate gullible young minds that what they see on television is not in their best interests. The total number of hours of television watched by children has been well charted. And the sponsors know when to make their pitch. It takes great willpower and strength for parents not to give in at the supermarket but instead to say 'no'. And bad habits can be hard to break!

It is our usual daily dietary habits that will help determine our general lifestyle and state of health. There is no doubt whatsoever about the long-term benefits of a diet that is high in protein, complex carbohydrates and vitamins, and low in fat, sugar and alcohol. Of course we will all weaken occasionally—and I am not advocating that we *never* eat take-away convenience food from time to time. But it must be the exception and not the rule. In battling CFS, and any other chronic condition for that matter, our bodies need all the help they can get!

Alternative therapies

Alternative therapies include:
- vitamin supplementation and anti-oxidant therapy
- herbal medicine
- homeopathy
- transcendental meditation.

Vitamin supplementation and anti-oxidants

For many years conventional medicine has frowned upon patients taking extra vitamins. We have always been told that, with an adequate and balanced diet, taking additional vitamins is unnecessary. There has never been any real scientific proof that vitamin therapy will help in treating the multitude of diseases for which it has become acclaimed.

My own feelings about vitamin therapy are coloured by my experience with patients and my own personal results. In short, I believe that the recommended daily allowance for most vitamins is far too low. Although not clinically proven, I sincerely believe that our need for vitamins varies, with a greater demand becoming necessary at times of stress (e.g. immune challenge due to infection).

Over the years I have treated many patients suffering from shingles—a painful, debilitating inflammation of nerve fibres caused by the latent herpes zoster virus becoming reactivated. It is the same virus that has previously caused chickenpox and that has remained dormant, usually for many years. The condition is always unilateral and characterised by a vesicular (blistery) rash that follows the course of a nerve. It frequently affects the chest wall but may occur elsewhere, including the face. If the ophthalmic division of the trigeminal nerve is involved, corneal scarring may occur, resulting in permanently impaired vision.

The development of the antiviral drug acyclovir has revolutionised the treatment of shingles. Provided treatment is commenced within the first few days of the appearance of the rash, the prognosis is excellent with usually complete resolution. In the days before acyclovir, the treatment was usually directed at relieving the pain of shingles with an appropriate analgesic and applying calamine lotion to the vesicles. In cases where sight was threatened oral steroids could be used, but there was nothing else available.

However, it was at the earliest possible time of treatment (i.e. at diagnosis) that I administered vitamin B12 by intramuscular injection twice weekly for several weeks. Over a period of twenty years, with no exceptions, my patients improved dramatically. The rash quickly subsided and there was little, if any, post-herpetic neuralgia. The only cases of shingles with complications that I ever saw were patients who had presented too late. They had been correctly diagnosed by another doctor but had not been given the benefits of vitamin B12 therapy. The results I obtained with vitamin B12 were almost as good as those obtained in later years with acyclovir; and when that became available I always gave patients the benefits of both.

I use this case to demonstrate my point. With the water-soluble vitamins (B group and C) there is little risk in using the bigger doses over a period of several weeks. They are excreted in the urine when not required, so cannot normally accumulate; although caution should be exercised with vitamin B6 (pyridoxine) and the mega-doses of vitamin C one sometimes reads about.

Vitamin C is the vitamin about which most claims have been made. It has been especially credited with strengthening the immune response and keeping common viruses (especially the cold and flu viruses) at bay. And it is frequently used as part of the treatment when one does succumb to these viruses. Doses used usually fall within the range of 250–1000 mg per day.

I believe that vitamin C in this dose range is harmless in most cases and very possibly beneficial as a prophylactic measure. Many patients swear by it and claim it helps to shorten the duration of their illness. Whether this is a 'placebo' effect or not, I must say I agree. Vitamin C is found in most fruits and vegetables and the minimum recommended daily allowance of 60 mg would be obtained from nearly every diet. Scurvy is seldom seen and is usually associated with sea voyages of centuries ago when fresh fruit was unobtainable. Alternately, mega-doses of more than 1000 mg a day could be harmful. Vitamin C can increase oxalate secretion in urine and could predispose to renal calculi. It is also thought to increase absorption of heavy metals (iron and aluminium), which could be damaging to both liver and brain.

The B group of vitamins are mostly water soluble and thought to aid in the immune response. They are helped in their absorption by vitamin C, which is frequently administered with them as a parenteral injection. B-group vitamins are found in a range of foods including milk, cheese, meats, fish, eggs and certain vegetables. Liver is a particularly rich source. The B-group vitamins are necessary for healthy skin, nerves and hair, and for many years have been implicated in the body's resistance to infection. Vitamin B6 (pyridoxine) is used in premenstrual tension but can cause nerve damage if taken in excess. Vitamin B12 deficiency usually occurs due to lack of absorption (and leads to pernicious anaemia) necessitating it being given by injection.

It is worth noting that both the B-group vitamins and vitamin C can be lost from our food by faulty cooking techniques. Vegetables should be steamed in a steaming basket within a lidded saucepan, or else simmered with minimal water. Alternately, they can be prepared easily by microwaving (again with minimal water) on the high setting for approximately four minutes.

Vitamin E, unlike the B group, is fat soluble. It is obtained from vegetable oils, nuts and dairy produce. It is available as a supplement (usually in a wheatgerm base), and moderate doses (250 mg) are thought to have a cardio-protective effect as well as preventing cell damage. Excessive amounts are unwise as it can raise blood triglyceride levels, lower thyroid gland hormones and actually worsen muscle weakness.

Over the last twenty years vitamin E has been credited with curing everything from impotence to premature ageing. But there is good reason to value vitamin E for its *anti-oxidant* qualities in which it is joined by vitamins A and C.

Free oxygen molecules are known to damage cells. Premature babies who are given oxygen at birth run the risk of damaged vision (due to retrolental fibroplasia) and are treated with vitamin E. In later life the role of oxidation in cell degeneration has been known for many years. It is thought that vitamin E (and A and C) neutralises the 'free radical' oxygen molecules and minimises the damage. It is often suggested that degenerative change, and ultimately all ageing, could therefore be slowed by using the anti-oxidant vitamins in a preventive way.

My experience with the anti-oxidant vitamins has been impressive. Patients of all ages have healed more quickly after surgery or traumatic wounds when given vitamins C and E in addition to a diet high in protein and complex carbohydrates. Many have felt so much better that they have remained on this anti-oxidant regimen; and their general health has been excellent, with very few suffering illnesses or conditions of a degenerative nature. In addition, this group of patients has had a conspicuously lower incidence of cardiovascular disease.

Another anti-oxidant often mentioned is carotene (vitamin A), found in carrots (especially), liver, green vegetables, eggs and milk. This is a fat-soluble vitamin that is stored in the body and which, if taken in high doses, is very definitely toxic. It can cause dry and pigmented skin, nausea and sore joints. It can also raise intra-cranial pressure. It is a vitamin so easily obtained in the diet that it should never need to be taken as a supplement.

So which vitamins should we take? A typical combination would be a simple multi-B group vitamin (there are many reliable brands) taken with 500 mg of vitamin C, and 250 mg of vitamin E (as alpha-tocopheryl acetate in a base of wheatgerm oil). At times of immunological stress, such as contact with infection or wound healing, the dosage of both the vitamin C and the vitamin E can be doubled. All these are widely available through chemists, health shops and supermarkets.

Of special relevance to CFS sufferers is the possible influence of anti-oxidants on reducing the influence of cytokines, which cause the symptoms. The cell damage that these chemicals cause at the neuromuscular junction would certainly be aggravated by oxygen 'free radicals', so I believe anti-oxidant vitamin therapy is justified. From a personal point of view I felt a considerable improvement in many of my symptoms after commencing on anti-oxidants on a daily basis, and I continue to take them to this day.

Herbal medicine

This is an area of alternative medicine that attracts a great deal of attention when conventional medicine does not have all the answers. Unfortunately it is also an area where both practitioners and therapies vary widely. Many herbalists are unqualified and some of their remedies have no scientific basis.

Because a drug is 'natural' does not make it harmless. Many of the most potent drugs in conventional medicine are derived from plants (e.g. digoxin) and the implications of dosage and side-effects are sometimes totally disregarded in the practice of herbal medicine.

Another worrying aspect is the free availability of these drugs. Many patients simply buy them at the health shop and self-administer, often with little knowledge of what they are taking. Possible long-term effects are not considered and, regrettably, many of these products have never been properly assessed in the first place.

Some of these drugs have quite devastating effects. A few are carcinogenic in laboratory animals, and others can adversely affect the body's hormone levels. Some are known to cause high blood pressure, while allergic reactions are probably much more common than we realise. In Australia recently there has been a death due to a hypersensitive reaction to Royal Jelly, a substance often recommended by alternative practitioners for its 'mysterious' qualities and healing properties for a diverse range of illnesses.

On the other hand, some natural remedies can be beneficial. Various teas are known to possess potent anti-oxidant qualities (see above) and evening primrose oil has been used to good effect in a variety of conditions from premenstrual tension to rheumatoid arthritis.

I would advise discussing any alternative therapies with your own doctor. He or she may certainly be sceptical and will probably be unfamiliar with many of the substances used in herbal medicine. But your doctor may also be aware of the possible side-effects and interactions with whatever other medication you may be taking.

Remember also the 'placebo' effect. Sometimes it is simply the thought that we are taking something 'special' that brings about some improvement. There is nothing wrong with this, of course; but if the 'something special' has a potentially dangerous long-term effect, then the whole exercise is extremely risky indeed (and probably very expensive as well).

There is something about chronic illnesses like CFS that makes the patient rather vulnerable. We are always on the lookout for that magic cure, constantly hoping that we will turn the corner. Positive thinking is very important and it is good to be optimistic. But that should not make the patient prey to those in the community who are out to make a 'fast buck'.

Homeopathy

Homeopathic medicine has been practised for more than a century and takes a holistic approach to both patients and their illnesses. In general, the preparations prescribed by a homeopath are made from natural sources and are used in diluted form to treat each patient on an individual basis.

The principle of homeopathy is to 'treat like with like'. In other words, the symptoms usually determine the treatment. Remedies are based on the patient's clinical presentation. If a healthy person were given the preparation they would probably suffer similar symptomatology. Yet in the patient who is already suffering those symptoms there is a reverse effect. Many CFS patients have derived some benefit from homeopathic medicine. Certainly there is no 'instant cure', but there can occur a lessening of some of the symptoms, which is what treatment is all about. As with several other alternative approaches, there is a place for homeopathy if other courses of action have failed.

Transcendental meditation

This technique of achieving total harmony of body and mind goes back thousands of years but has been revived to good effect over the last 30 years. There are now many schools that teach TM and it has become a valuable adjunct to conventional medicine in the treatment of many modern-day illnesses.

Meditation has its origins in Eastern civilisation but it can be practised to good effect whatever one's religion or cultural identity. Its aim is to allow the active thinking mind to drift in an unbounded, restful yet alert state by which we reach a higher level of consciousness than we would otherwise experience. We 'transcend' thinking in order to achieve a purer and less distracted consciousness. This process of restoring harmony to the mind results in a greatly relaxed and natural homeostasis of the body's physiology.

The benefits of TM are both physiological and psychological. The implications in a clinical setting are significant, with far-reaching benefits to many medical conditions, not just those that are stress related. These results are being increasingly recognised by the medical profession, albeit slowly, with the realisation that meditation may even replace medication in some situations. It's for good reason that major insurance companies in the USA and parts of Europe offer significant bonuses to clients who routinely meditate.

The physiological benefits are numerous. There occurs a decreased respiration rate, blood pressure and heart rate, with a corresponding decrease in oxygen consumption and metabolic rate. There is a sharp increase in skin resistance (indicating a better response to stress) and changes in electroencephalogram patterns (EEG), which confirm a restful alertness. There is an increased production of serotonin and a lowered amount of adrenalin. Both cortisol and cholesterol levels are reduced and the immune response is improved.

Psychological benefits include a decreased incidence of both anxiety and depressive disorders. There is a reduced reliance upon drugs and alcohol, and an improved sleeping pattern. Personality disorders and aggression are less frequent, combined with an improved ability to cope. Learning capabilities and IQ are also improved, as are motor and perceptual skills.

Interestingly, most of these changes can be proven. It is very simple to show the improved physiological parameters in a group who practise TM compared with a control group. And the benefits to a multitude of medical conditions are obvious. Even the ageing process is slowed in those who include TM as part of their daily routine. Many look (and feel) years younger.

TM is becoming an increasingly important part of managing cardiovascular disease in those patients prepared to try it. Its beneficial effect in lowering blood pressure has been well documented, and its cholesterol-lowering effect is extremely significant although the mechanism of action remains unclear. Patients who meditate regularly also find it easier to give up cigarette smoking (and other substance abuse).

The benefits to the immune response are especially relevant for CFS sufferers. The changes that occur at a chemical (neurotransmitter) level will help to counteract many of the most debilitating symptoms. TM should be seriously considered as an important part of any treatment regimen.

It is not difficult to learn the technique of TM. The sooner you learn and start practising regularly, the more benefits will occur, to both body and mind. Most often the technique is taught in classes or groups; and then an individual session is usual where a personalised *mantra* (a key word or phrase) is issued to the person.

Most techniques will focus attention on breathing, reducing muscle tension, listening and the use of the mantra. It is important to practise TM in a quiet place with little risk of interruption. Taking the phone off the hook or leaving the answering machine on is advisable. It is recommended that you practise TM for twenty minutes twice daily—before breakfast and dinner is suitable—for maximum benefit, although the technique can be applied at any time of the day or night.

It is best to adopt a sitting position with the back and neck straight. Lying down is also possible but the aim is not to go to sleep. The position should be relaxed with no obvious muscle tension. Gently close the eyes and breathe in slowly and deeply. Allow the thoughts to come and go without dwelling on any particular thought or subject. With the out breath, allow the muscles to relax and the tension to dissipate.

Be aware of the body's presence in the chair with the arms of the chair supporting your upper limbs. Allow the breathing to fall into a normal, natural rhythm with any particular thoughts put out of your mind. Be aware of your neck and shoulder and let any tension melt away. Then feel the weight of your arms falling away. Feel your body weight on the chair as you move your attention to the thighs and legs. If tension should remain, then practise letting it go as you maintain your posture with a minimum effort.

Be aware of your breathing. In fact allow your attention to settle on the breaths you take. Don't fight any thought or images that superimpose themselves. Allow them to pass as freely as they came. Don't give them your attention. Instead refocus on the breathing and remain detached from any distracting images in the mind. Feel yourself becoming immune to any stray thought that may enter your mind.

Listen to sounds in the distance. Don't dwell on them or they will become thoughts. Just be aware of them as you rest. Practise letting go of any thoughts, no matter what they might be.

Think of your word (mantra) and repeat it in your mind when you feel the need to eliminate other thoughts. Use it as an anchor and come back to it if your mind starts to wander. Remember, it is your mantra and should be used each time you meditate. Repeat it again and again (in your mind) and let it transport you into the realms where you have transcended normal levels of awareness.

When it is time to descend from your state of peaceful, undisturbed consciousness, let your eyes open slowly. Become aware of your immediate surroundings as you feel your muscles starting to move again. Slowly move your arms and legs and feel your body renewed, and your mind relaxed.

During TM the body can often rest more in minutes than we sometimes achieve in hours of sleep. The benefits to total body physiology and restorative powers are obvious. It is for good reason that TM has its wide and dedicated following. With continued practice and incorporation into your lifestyle, the benefits to treatment of any chronic disorder, including CFS, are immense.

TM does not suit everyone. Even among those who extol its virtues, the results vary greatly. However, for people with a long-term illness who regularly practise TM there is often a marked improvement in their ability to cope with their illness, regardless of whether or not they notice any physiological benefits as well.

Spinal decompression surgery

The results of surgically relieving the pressure in suitably selected patients with severe cervical stenosis or Chiari malformation appear impressive.

Data presented by Chicago neurosurgeon Dr Dan Heffez

at a meeting of the National Fibromyalgia Research Association (USA) in 1999 revealed that, of a severely affected group who underwent surgery, nearly 100 per cent of those suffering headaches, disorientation, sleeping difficulties and peripheral numbness showed improvement or complete resolution of the problem up to six months after surgery. More than 75 per cent of those with irritable bowel syndrome, short-term memory, concentration difficulties or visual problems had improved or were normal up to six months after surgery. And more than 60 per cent saw improvement or resolution of muscle weakness or fatigue within the same period.

Much more research is needed to establish the incidence of spinal cord compression before neurosurgery can be considered as part of the tratment of CFS or fibromyalgia. And many of those with cervical stenosis are not severely enough affected to justify such surgical intervention. For these patients, Dr Heffez would recommend less invasive treatments such as wearing a cervical collar, posture training and a brief course of steroids (for no longer than a week) to reduce inflammation.

Case studies

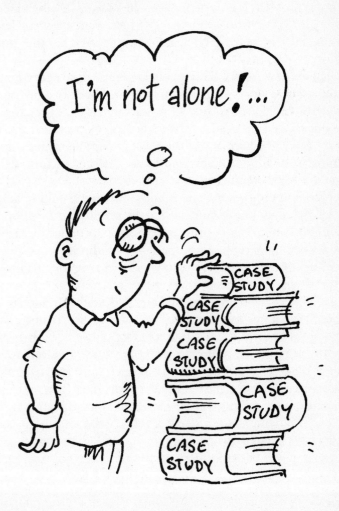

During my years in general practice I treated a number of patients who were suffering from CFS. Since my illness, with the benefits of hindsight, I sometimes wonder if there had been others. The rather diverse symptoms can bring about a varying clinical picture which, to put it mildly, can be a diagnostic dilemma. It was especially so in the days before CFS became a recognised condition.

My knowledge of CFS was limited to what I had read in the journals. Certainly it was never taught about at medical school. Nor was it ever mentioned, although we were made aware of 'post-viral syndromes' where patients were left drained of all energy. The usual outcome was that they got better — eventually!

The most typical CFS patients were previously fit young adults. Their illness could often be traced back to a definite infectious episode that had knocked them about more than was usual and left them in a weakened state. I suspect there may well have been more than one infectious agent and, almost certainly, one or more of the 'trigger factors' discussed earlier in this book.

Like a jigsaw puzzle, the missing pieces are falling into place. We now know more about the syndrome. There is a definition, and ongoing research that has produced clearer guidelines when evaluating a patient's condition.

Many of the patients remain vividly clear in my memory. I know that most made a complete recovery, and several have gone on to pursue active careers despite the interruptions necessitated by their illnesses. I also realise, thankfully, that I did everything possible as a supportive GP to help them through their suffering, although I was frustrated by there being no specific cure available. And yet my own experiences over the past couple of years have given me an immeasurably greater empathy with all of them.

The following cases include several of my own patients. They have been happy to share their stories in the hope that more light will be thrown on this mysterious syndrome. The remaining case histories are of patients I have met since

becoming one of them. Likewise, they realise the importance of CFS research and are eager to help with their own
personal experiences. My thanks go to all of them.

JANE R, aged 38, was a career woman. She had been involved
in the world of finance since obtaining a commerce degree at
the University of Melbourne. She was now based in New York,
but her work involved frequent air travel to other places and, as
she once aptly remarked, she lived most of her time out of a
suitcase. She had both business and social contacts in Melbourne and returned at least twice a year.

She was great fun to be with and had a wide circle of friends.
She tended to save up any medical problems until she returned
home to Australia, and would always visit me for routine medical checks, gynaecological Pap smears and any necessary pre-
scriptions. I had been her GP for about twelve years and always
looked forward to her cheerful smile.

On this particular occasion, however, I could hardly believe
my eyes as I ushered her from the waiting room into my office.
She looked drained, pale and years older. Her bubbling chatter
was less effervescent and her smile was more a strained
attempt at recognition. I knew she had difficulty walking and
her once sprightly jaunt had become a slow, unsteady gait.

Jane gave a two-month history of increasing tiredness. She
had been on holiday in the Caribbean and had been ill with a
form of gastroenteritis. This persisted for almost a week,
necessitating her early return to New York. Her doctor diagnosed a viral infection and recommended that she convalesce
at home before returning to work. The symptoms settled and
she resumed her fairly frantic lifestyle within a fortnight. But the
tiredness persisted and she started to complain of muscle pain,
headaches and a disturbance in short-term memory. She was
particularly worried by the latter and, half jokingly, asked if it
could be early Alzheimer's disease.

Further questioning revealed a fairly typical story of a definite
infectious episode followed by a period of fatigue aggravated by
exercise and only partially helped by rest. Although the initial

gastroenteritis symptoms had disappeared, she actually felt worse than ever. She was frankly frightened by this strange exhaustion and felt threatened by her inability to resume her normal routine.

My examination of Jane revealed no other abnormalities. In particular, a neurological examination was normal and there was no evidence of muscle wasting. Routine tests of the blood and the urine were arranged, and Jane was advised to rest until the results came through.

A few days later I saw Jane again, but not in the surgery. Her muscle weakness had prevented her coming to me, so a home visit was arranged instead. She welcomed me at the door and looked better than at her first visit to me several days earlier. The bed rest had done some good.

By the time of my second visit, I was already certain of the diagnosis. The largely unremarkable results of the pathology tests had excluded some very important treatable conditions, so I felt more confident in labelling Jane's illness as CFS.

My patient treated the news with mixed feelings. She was obviously glad that nothing more serious had been revealed. But she knew enough about CFS from having lived in the USA to recognise that it was a debilitating condition that could persist for a long time. There were important implications for her work and she tended to be concerned about that above all else.

Jane accepted both my diagnosis and advice. Over the next month she arranged to take leave from her organisation for a period of six months and to stay in Melbourne where she had friends, family and support. She also accepted the rather uncertain outlook and was prepared to do everything required to regain her health as soon as possible.

After six months there was some improvement. Jane was able to walk a small distance every day and was remarkably astute at recognising her limits. Forever the organiser, she had arranged her flat to suit her needs and a small army of friends were only too ready to help her if required. But like so many CFS sufferers, including myself, she valued her independence and relied on outside help only when absolutely necessary.

There was no way Jane could fully resume her career at this stage. She had kept in touch and was fully computer literate, which was a great advantage. But for her the number of working hours per day was still very limited, and she knew the dangers of extending herself beyond her given energy levels. Her employers were very understanding and obviously had insight into her condition. It was they who suggested she remain in Australia for as long as need be and they rearranged her work load so that it became manageable.

The following twelve months saw Jane improve steadily. Of course she had her remissions and her exacerbations. She knew the frustration that is common to all CFS patients when she was prevented from doing something that anyone else would have taken for granted. But with each remission there was a sturdier platform from which to function. Small tasks became possible and, with systematic organisation, Jane set herself a realistic time frame in which to get better.

In many ways Jane was a model patient. She changed her dietary habits to comply with those principles outlined in Chapter 5. She kept in touch with friends by phone and never allowed her illness to cause them to lose contact. She joined a voluntary support group whose many CFS sufferers were battling to come to terms with their illness. And she never once entertained the notion that she would become a long-term victim of CFS. Although at times depressed, she mostly thought positively throughout that period and was able to see the light at the end of the tunnel.

After a convalescence of eighteen months, Jane resumed her career. She had remained in touch with her management firm throughout the long months of her illness. She certainly modified her commitments and took on a less demanding schedule. But at least she was leading a so-called 'normal existence'.

When I last spoke to Jane she was engaged. She rang to tell me the news, and had heard about my own experience. She still has occasional warning symptoms and has to slow down if she becomes tired. But she has learned to obey her body. In doing so she has achieved control over her CFS, rather than letting it control her.

MATTHEW P was just fourteen years old when his mother brought him to see me. The family had moved to Melbourne from interstate as a result of Matthew's father being transferred by his firm some six months earlier. Mrs P was worried by Matthew's frequent 'off' days, during which he just wanted to lie down. He had missed several weeks of school and was getting behind in his class. His primary symptom was tiredness, with little else to report.

Matthew looked a bright and healthy boy. He spoke quietly and thought deeply before responding to my questions. He gave intelligent answers and was able to give a good history, with minimal interjection from his mother, who looked more tired and anxious than he did.

I had looked after Mrs P's family for many years. She was originally from Melbourne and her sister's children were all patients as well. Her mother was still alive and robust at the age of 93, and her father, who had founded one of Melbourne's leading law firms, had died of prostatic cancer some years earlier.

According to Mrs P, Matthew was having one of his better days. In fact he had been brought directly from school, where he had spent his first half-day in over four weeks. By looks alone, he appeared as healthy as any other fourteen-year-old. But, as I was soon to learn, Matthew had been running on 'half charge' for months.

Soon after settling into his new school, Matthew started to complain of frequent fatigue. 'He's always tired,' volunteered his mother, 'even first thing in the morning.' Matthew nodded in agreement, adding that his teachers had frequently noticed it as well. One master thought he had a behavioural problem, and another had accused him of not paying attention. Even the other boys had nick-named him 'dopey', which hadn't helped a bit.

Matthew had always been a bright child. He frequently topped the class at his previous school and was good at games and sports. He made model aeroplanes and learned to play the flute—so well, in fact, that he was in demand to play at the school's concerts. He was popular with the other children and had always enjoyed school enormously. He had seldom been ill, other than a tendency to develop tonsillitis and occasional middle-ear infections.

Matthew was the youngest of three children. His older sister had commenced university studies and his brother was a boarder at secondary school level. Being the only one at home was not a problem for Matthew, and he seemed to have coped well with transferring from his previous school, although it meant leaving most of his friends and starting in a new environment. Importantly he had never shown any tendency to be a malingerer.

It was the change of schools that Mrs P blamed for Matthew's symptoms. She had discussed the problem with one of his teachers, who was also concerned about the boy's fatigue. And yet Matthew was not overdoing it. He enjoyed his limited sport; and he was still performing reasonably well in class, although his grades had slipped from excellent to just average. Bedtime was strictly adhered to and Mrs P made sure he had a healthy, adequate diet. She felt sure it was the result of changing schools, but, after talking it through with his head teacher, decided to bring Matthew in for assessment.

It appeared that the symptoms had commenced soon after Matthew started at his new school. Apart from being constantly tired, Matthew had suffered from occasional headaches and pain in his muscles, which for him was most unusual. He noticed that sport made his symptoms worse and that reading for lengthy periods made his eyes ache and produced some visual disturbance, as did sitting too far back in class.

His concentration was also poor. His family had noticed that his attention span had decreased, and he frequently seemed listless and unhappy. Even small excursions and minimal efforts, both physical and mental, made him exhausted. Sleeping patterns were not good and appetite was sporadic.

Physical examination was basically normal. His weight was in the lower range for his height and he had several enlarged submandibular lymph nodes in the neck. There was a low-grade inflammation of the throat but no sign of any ear infection. His sight, in particular, was excellent with no decrease in visual activity.

I arranged some blood tests and a paediatric opinion. Although CFS went through my mind I did not mention it at that stage, but recommended that Matthew rest at home until we reviewed the results. Most of his troublesome symptoms subsided very quickly on bed rest, which I felt was also an indication of CFS.

Matthew's paediatrician had a good knowledge of CFS in children. He had diagnosed the condition in several children who had presented with a more diverse clinical picture, but in whom fatigue was a predominant symptom. So I had confidence in his opinion and was not surprised when he confirmed my suspicion. He agreed that Matthew should continue his period of rest for several more weeks, and then gradually increase his mobility. He was to have several periods a day of walking on flat ground and hydrotherapy at a local heated pool twice a week. My recommended diet, high in protein and complex carbohydrates, was endorsed. And very little medication was advised other than a multi B-group vitamin supplement and paracetamol if necessary for the muscle pain.

Matthew made excellent progress at home. It was six months before he felt strong enough to cope with the demands of school, and even then he went for only half a normal school day for another two months. During his period at home he was able to do a little school work in several sessions a day. There was seldom a day when he was unable to do anything, and the energy levels gradually returned to normal.

Matthew's school teachers were a great help in his recovery. Once they understood the diagnosis they arranged for him to do a limited amount of syllabus work which, to begin with, was a trial-and-error affair. Some days were obviously better than others, but over the six-month period there was sufficient improvement to allow a graduated and supervised return to school. There was full expectation that Matthew would have to repeat the year, but, as it turned out, this was not necessary; nor was child counselling, which was considered at one stage.

The understanding and cooperation between parents and teachers of a child with CFS is of vital importance. The potential for a major disruption to the child's education is great. However, it can be minimised by having a definite diagnosis at the earliest stage, and by accepting its implications and making the most of what can be offered to the child in terms of school and community support.

MRS LYNNE B was 42 years old and the mother of two boys aged ten and twelve. Her husband worked in an insurance company. The family seemed happy and well adjusted. There had been problems of a financial nature earlier in their marriage, but these had apparently been resolved.

Lynne was a healthy and energetic woman with lots of interests. Although her family was her main preoccupation she involved herself in several community projects and was an active member of her local church group. She had been a teacher before her marriage but had no desire to return to work, believing that a mother's place was in the home.

Over the years, I had come to know the family well. Both sons had their normal share of childhood ailments and the occasional laceration that needed sutures. One child was also asthmatic but this was well controlled with maintenance therapy. So it was unusual to see Lynne without her usual entourage as I called her in from the waiting room.

The normally robust 42-year-old sat in front of me looking tired and drawn. She proceeded to list her symptoms and her tale of increasing inability to keep up with her normal activities.

Lynne had never been ill since I'd known her. Both her pregnancies were uncomplicated and she had no significant family history of illness. She had taken no medication since ceasing the oral contraceptive pill two years previously when her husband had decided to undergo a vasectomy.

Her present problem had started about a month earlier. There was no definite viral-type illness of which she was aware. Instead, she suffered a severe throbbing unilateral headache behind one eye. Associated with this was photophobia and eye strain that lasted beyond the headache and was further aggravated by reading or close work. About the same time, she noticed joint pains and aching muscles, aggravated by minimal physical exertion and relieved by rest. Her sleeping pattern was also disturbed and she inevitably woke feeling just as tired as when she went to bed. Libido was poor and she was unable to concentrate for any length of time.

Further questioning revealed the symptom that upset her the most. Overwhelming fatigue had been a constant complaint even when the other symptoms had lessened. For a person as active as Lynne this was the worst aspect of all. She was having trouble with the most simple domestic duties and at times even questioned her own sanity. She was not depressed, but anxiety and frustration were starting to disrupt her life as never before.

Following an uneventful examination, blood tests and a cerebral scan were organised. These showed a borderline anaemia consistent with iron deficiency, but were otherwise normal. As Lynne's menstrual periods were light and regular it was possible that her diet might be lacking in some way. She then confessed that, at times, she had even been too tired to get up for proper meals. It took all her energy just to perform the minimal tasks. She would prepare the evening meal for her family and go back to bed.

When I was sure of the diagnosis I arranged to see both Lynne and her husband. He was keen to help and was obviously a vital part of Lynne's support network. We discussed the ways we could help some of her symptoms and the changes that would need to be made in the running of the household.

Rest was obviously the most immediate part of Lynne's treatment. She would need assistance in the house to take care of normal household duties, plus someone to shop and cook for the family. Her husband was reassuring in this regard and had already made enquiries through a neighbour about regular home help. The two boys were old enough to appreciate the situation and they too were a great help in their mother's convalescence.

The following three months were difficult for Lynne. She had accepted that she was unable to do most of what she was accustomed to doing, but felt strangely helpless when bed-bound. However, with a supervised diet, plenty of rest and the use of anti-inflammatory drugs there was a great deal of improvement, even after just three months.

When the three months were up we increased Lynne's mobilisation. There were obviously 'bad' days when not much could be achieved. But at other times it was possible to introduce a graded program of walks and the lightest of tasks around the home. The daily help was an immense relief—and a revelation just how much many wives and mothers are really worth, and how we tend to take them for granted!

It was another eighteen months before Lynne improved to the point of not needing outside help. By this time her husband and sons had worked out an excellent routine. The household was running smoothly, groceries were delivered several times a week, and Lynne was able to supervise many of their require-ments over the phone. She was still having muscle problems, but the sleeping pattern and short-term memory had returned to normal. Headaches were less frequent and the vision prob-lems had resolved.

By a strange turn of events, Lynne is now a counsellor with a CFS support group. We have spoken several times and, for a change, she has given me advice. It is five years since her ill-ness began and she has almost recovered completely. The remissions have lasted longer, and the relapses have been less frequent and certainly less severe. She has learned the crucial knack of 'pacing' herself, and her lifestyle, as a result, has been suitably adapted.

DR RICHARD M was a dentist aged 35 when I first met him at a lecture given by a CFS support group in Sydney. He had developed CFS three years earlier and was by now over the worst of his illness. His story struck me as an ideal case history, because he had suffered several quite diverse medical problems before finally being diagnosed.

Like many in his profession, Richard worked long hours. He also played hard, and spent his weekends either sailing, playing tennis or working on a hobby farm he had bought and improved with a view to growing grapevines.

Richard first presented to his doctor with a typical case of glandular fever. He had a ten-day history of a sore throat, enlarged glands and profound fatigue. He confessed to his GP that he had already taken a course of antibiotics in the hope that they would knock the infection as quickly as possible. Instead, they had been of no use at all and Richard felt as ill as ever.

Aware of the fact that many dentists and doctors can be terrible patients, his GP made him promise to rest in bed until he received the results of some blood tests. Richard agreed, too exhausted to do otherwise. His wife (of just six months) decided to stay home from her part-time work to look after him. There were no children in the family.

The results came through as infectious mononucleosis and confirmed the doctor's suspicion. Richard took over a month to improve to the point where he could gradually resume his work. On his GP's advice, he halved his sessions and cut out all social engagements for a further month. At the end of that time he appeared to have fully recovered and felt well enough to resume full-time work.

It was two months later when Richard made an appointment to see his GP again. He said he had felt well for the first month and had then started to notice muscle pain on climbing the stairs at work. There followed a period of several hours during which he felt totally exhausted, similar to when he was ill with glandular fever. He had also become forgetful and had difficulty sleeping at night. His weekend activities had been cancelled and he remained in bed to help cope with the myalgia and fatigue. Other symptoms included headaches, nausea, abdominal pain and a marked intolerance to alcohol.

Richard's clinical presentation was highly suggestive of CFS. The earlier viral infection (glandular fever) followed by the fatigue, myalgia, cerebral symptoms and associated gastrointestinal disturbances all pointed to that diagnosis. But at that stage his GP, who was unfamiliar with CFS, felt it was necessary to exclude certain other conditions.

Because of the prominence of cerebral symptoms, Richard was at first investigated neurologically. A thorough examination threw no new light on the cause of his illness and a brain scan was normal. Meanwhile, at only 32 years of age and an early stage in his career, Richard was becoming more and more depressed with no improvement in sight. He readily agreed to his GP's suggestion that he see another specialist physician.

Richard was finally diagnosed as having CFS, but the physician was sufficiently concerned by his abdominal symptoms to organise a gastroscopy. This showed no ulcer or growth, but instead established the presence of a diffuse gastritis. Subsequent pathology tests on the samples taken revealed an infection with *Helicobacter pylori*. It was difficult to say how long he had been infected. Fortunately, a combination of antibacterial drugs solved this problem, and his abdominal symptoms soon resolved.

Unfortunately there was no such positive effect on his other symptoms. Muscle fatigue was the most limiting problem and sometimes even minimal exertion brought on profound exhaustion. Simple tasks became major obstacles and a short walk often left Richard feeling as though he had run a mile.

The headaches were unlike migraine, but were severe and seemingly independent of anything in his diet that might have triggered them. He reluctantly took the analgesics advised by his doctor, but felt that they exaggerated his mental fogginess and worsened his daytime sleepiness.

Richard was indeed mentally 'foggy' and forgetful, and he had considerable difficulty sleeping at night. Not only was it difficult getting to sleep, but he frequently woke during the night and sometimes couldn't get back to sleep, especially if the muscle pain was present as well. Most mornings he woke feeling as tired as ever and he tended to sleep most of the day as a result.

As a result of the diagnosis, Richard had to rearrange his life. He accepted that he must adjust his priorities and acknowledge his limits. He gave up any hope of working in the immediate future and used what little energy he had in pursuing every book and journal dealing with CFS. His colleagues showed little understanding of his illness and suggested that he was probably having some type of breakdown. Such ignorance did not help, but was fortunately counterbalanced by the increasing awareness of CFS in the community and the knowledge that it was becoming the subject of research, both at home and abroad.

The following twelve months saw Richard becoming increasingly attracted to alternative medicine. He tried herbal remedies, yoga and acupuncture, all with little result. A prevailing theory among the dental profession was that the mercury in dental amalgam could be a factor in CFS. So several fillings were replaced—again to no real avail.

Adapting his lifestyle and knowing his limits had at least minimised the symptoms as much as possible. The treatment Richard feels helped him most was dietary modification combined with a carefully graded exercise program and transcendental meditation. The latter certainly helped him to cope with the situation and may well have had a more direct effect on the levels of chemical neurotransmitters in his body.

His diet and mobilisation were crucial adaptations for the better. The diet, which was high in protein and complex carbohydrates and low in fats and sugar, helped to stabilise his energy levels. The exercise program mobilised the muscles and joints in a gradual and gentle way. And the judicious use of an anti-inflammatory drug and a tricyclic antidepressant helped reduce the severity of the symptoms.

The support Richard received from friends and family helped him to get through the most debilitating periods of CFS. He was also encouraged by the large number of patients who kept in touch by contacting him at home (and I can vouch for how therapeutic that can be!). His wife's adaptation of his bedroom into a communication centre with phone, fax and personal computer meant that he had access to the outside world and could remain in touch when his symptoms were at their worst.

After a further eighteen months, Richard returned to part-time dentistry. He is still limited in what he can achieve physically but, with care, he is making steady progress. The frustration and depression are gone, the muscle pains are controlled and the fatigue is kept to a minimum by Richard's technique of pacing himself. Optimism has replaced despair as he goes forth with the worst of his CFS behind him, and a realistic attitude to life.

SALLY W, a mother of two, had just turned 46. Her daughter was completing a degree in architecture and her son was training to be a pilot. Both were in their early twenties and were starting to lead very independent lives. It had been a close family, saddened only by the sudden death of Sally's husband ten years earlier in a car accident.

I met Sally socially. Our mutual host knew we had both been diagnosed with CFS and probably had a lot in common. The self-assured woman appeared the picture of health, her bright eyes and flawless complexion gave no indication that she was battling with CFS. (But then, I myself had been complimented on how well I looked, so I understood how deceptive appearances can be.)

Like me, Sally had endured more than a year of constant, debilitating ill health, and was at last having sufficient remissions to re-establish a few semblances of a normal existence. As we were meeting socially on equal terms, without the boundaries of a doctor–patient contract, we were both eager to 'compare notes'.

Sally's illness came on suddenly. It had started three years earlier following an attack of gastroenteritis which, she suspected, was 'caught' in hospital. Heavy and irregular periods had led to a hysterectomy for a fibroid uterus. The operation itself was a complete success, but on the day of her discharge she developed diarrhoea and vomiting.

The gastroenteritis was treated at home by her GP. Within two or three days the symptoms had settled, but Sally remained weak and tired. In particular, she noticed severe muscle fatigue that seemed out of all proportion to the trivial physical exertion that precipitated it.

To complicate matters, Sally developed headaches, night sweats and a frustrating disturbance in short-term memory. These symptoms appeared within days of her discharge from hospital and her GP was initially concerned about post-operative complications. However, it was ten days since her surgery, there was no localised sign of infection and the wound was healing nicely. The gynaecologist called to see her at home and could find nothing abnormal on pelvic examination. After discussing the symptoms with her GP, she was re-admitted for further investigations.

Back in hospital Sally underwent a series of blood tests, urine cultures, chest and pelvic X-rays, and scans of her abdomen and brain. The only abnormalities found were some atypical lymphocytes on the blood film. Her night sweats subsided and the headaches became less severe. The exhaustion was not so obvious either, as she was mostly in bed. By the time of her discharge from hospital a week later, the symptoms were labelled as 'post-viral' and she was reassured that nothing serious had been found.

Sally's muscle fatigue soon re-emerged as her major symptom. She was at home alone and was unable to rest quite as much as she had in hospital. Nevertheless, she spent nearly all her time lying down, getting up only for meals and to shower each morning. In fact the effort of showering and making her bed would sometimes exhaust her so much that there was no option but to return to bed.

The other reason for returning to bed so frequently was her excessive sleepiness. Even in the mornings, after a full night's sleep, she was often tired and unrefreshed. She had always thrived on six or seven hours' sleep. Now she needed at least twelve hours' sleep every night and frequent naps during the day as well.

Sally blamed this hypersomnia for her foggy mentality. Indeed, her concentration and short-term memory had never been so bad, and she even had trouble finding her words at times. This problem fluctuated depending on what she had been doing and was usually worse after prolonged mental activity like reading or watching a movie.

I listened to Sally in amazement. Many of these symptoms were so familiar. In particular, I could identify with the muscle fatigue, the exhaustion, the sleep disturbances and the mental fogginess. We both agreed how the severity of the symptoms could fluctuate, even throughout the course of a single day.

Sally explained how she underwent further tests. Her GP had referred her to a specialist in infectious diseases who ran a series of serology tests, as well as checking her for thyroid, rheumatoid and metabolic disorders. His final verdict came as a shock to Sally, but not to her daughter Lisa, who had returned home to help look after her mother. Lisa had suspected CFS from the outset, as one of her favourite tutors had been struck down with it and she was familiar with many of the symptoms.

The next twelve months saw Sally reorganise her life and face a period of uncertainty and inactivity. She was determined to get better, but all the positive thinking in the world did not make the symptoms less troublesome. But CFS was at least being recognised and she was able to learn about its management and the developments that were happening overseas. She had also heard of various medical teams studying CFS in Australia, despite a lack of government funding.

Prior to Sally's illness she was on the point of becoming engaged. She had been widowed for seven years and, now that her children were grown up, she was tempted by the companionship that a second marriage would offer. She was still only 43 when diagnosed with CFS. So there was an added incentive to get over this debilitating illness.

Her fiancé was totally supportive throughout the two years that followed. He had been divorced some years earlier and was looking forward to a new chapter in both their lives.

Sally's progress in getting over CFS did not gain pace until the end of her second year with the illness. She was still limited, especially by the muscle fatigue and the need for extra sleep. She was depressed at times, but considered this to be normal. Her concentration and memory returned to normal after one year, and the headaches were much less troublesome. Symptoms of irritable bowel syndrome were prone to occur if she strayed too much from her diet (which coincided very much with my diet outlined in Chapter 5), and she still had a marked intolerance to alcohol.

The last six months had been the best. She was able to walk for a reasonable distance each day and her sleeping pattern was not as abnormal as it had been. She had learned to pace her activities and she put her limited energy reserves to good use. She was even able to enjoy a little gardening. And, happily, she was planning their wedding to take place the following autumn. CFS or not, life must go on.

MRS MARY K is an intelligent woman in her early sixties. Her academic achievements included an Arts degree from the University of Melbourne. She also had a Diploma of Education, was a qualified librarian, and had published one book on local history as well as being involved in two more. She admitted to being a perfectionist, which was obvious from her books and from the computerised medical history she had prepared for me.

Mary had been diagnosed as suffering from CFS eight years earlier. But her medical problems went back further. She was in her mid-thirties when she contracted glandular fever. At that time she had been married ten years and was bringing up three young children. She had lost a baby shortly after birth, and another was stillborn. Perhaps only partly aware of it at the time, she never got over those infant deaths, and her grief would remain unresolved for many years. Her illness occurred within a short time of the family returning home from the United Kingdom and the USA, where her husband had been sent on a study scholarship for a year or so. Her progress was complicated by a post-viral syndrome, which eventually subsided.

At that stage of her life, Mary was extraordinarily energetic. She not only ran the home and brought up three children, but managed to teach English part-time at a girls' college. When she was unable to continue her teaching commitments, she obtained a job in the library of the school where her husband taught and set about gaining her library qualifications in what spare time remained.

Looking back now, more than twenty years later, Mary admits she was doing too much. In addition to raising her children, part-time work and spare-time study, there were other family responsibilities. Her parents were elderly and developing health problems. They were a further demand on her time and energy. Within a few years she fell ill, with symptoms of a viral upper-respiratory infection. A disturbing feature was that the aches and pains (especially affecting her neck and shoulders) lasted nine months. However, she still managed to pass her library examinations with honours and eventually returned to full-time work.

The next few years saw pressures increase both at home and at work. She had a hysterectomy for a fibroid uterus, and reacted badly to the anaesthetic. After her mother's death, her father became increasingly senile, requiring more care and eventually institutionalisation. Later that same year, Mary suffered another major illness characterised by sore throat, swollen glands and muscular fatigue. The symptoms again lasted about nine months, after which she returned to work. But the changes at work, with computerisation, made it increasingly difficult to cope. She became anxious and developed sleep problems, leading to her resignation at the age of 52.

Mary made good use of her retirement. She became involved in writing and took up golf, which she greatly enjoyed. Dressmaking was another hobby, and she now had more time to socialise and catch up with old friends. She also looked forward to another trip to England with her husband. This unfortunately was marred by further episodes of muscular pains and fatigue and, on her return to Australia, she was diagnosed (for the first time) as suffering from CFS, or ME (myalgic encephalomyelitis) as it was then commonly termed.

Various avenues were explored to treat Mary's 'new' illness. The common analgesics caused constipation and nausea, and all the anti-inflammatory drugs upset her stomach. Her muscle pains were helped greatly by Chinese acupuncture, but herbal treatments were not of much use. Her diet was important, and she made every effort to avoid foods to which she had developed an allergy. She also received psychological counselling to help deal with the unresolved grief over the infant deaths from years earlier, which had been revived somewhat with the arrival of her first grandchild.

Mary takes very little regular medication, and none specifically for CFS. A gastric pre-ulcer condition was diagnosed, for which she takes the occasional course of ranitidine (a drug that decreases the production of stomach acid) when troubled by abdominal pain. She has also continued to take hormone replacement therapy, like many other women of her age. And she uses trifluoperazine (an anti-anxiety drug) occasionally, if she feels excessively stressed or tense.

Mary's CFS could be described as in remission, but liable to recur in certain circumstances. She has become astute at recognising the early symptoms of a relapse. There is usually a groggy feeling in the head and behind the eyes, together with an abnormal tongue sensation. These are usually followed by a weakness of the legs and an overwhelming sense of fatigue. She then notices aching limbs and joints, soreness and tightness of the throat, dry and itchy eyes, and a feeling of depression.

Mary also feels her age is a complicating factor. Some of her symptoms she could well attribute to 'getting on a bit', especially the limb and joint pains. She certainly thinks the ageing process has made it harder to deal with CFS, and she has developed a fairly rigid daily regimen in order to prevent relapses. After being up and down 'like a see-saw' for the first eighteen months, her CFS has now been fairly stable for six years.

The factors that precipitated a relapse were also predictable. Inadequate sleep, prolonged stress (including anxiety, excitement, or even concentration) and an irregular or poor diet (with possible allergies or reactions to preservatives and other chemicals) were all implicated. Mary also stressed the importance of a correct balance of exercise and rest, and the avoidance of sudden drops or extremes of temperature.

Her typical day follows a pattern. She is a 'morning person' and, unlike most CFS sufferers, is actually at her best early in the day. It is during the morning that she performs most of her tasks, including study and computer work. Although reading and writing are important to her, she limits these activities to an hour at a time. She also enjoys small amounts of shopping, walking and gardening, if possible. She tries to be home by 12.30 p.m. and, after lunch, lies down for about two hours. She may sleep for about an hour or do some relaxation exercises.

Mary has a small but close network of friends who understand her limitations. She would like to be able to play tennis or golf, but avoids the temptation. Any extra physical stress can be risky, and she has even had problems blowing up a child's party balloon. Although she is unable to attend luncheons, she keeps in touch with her friends. Evening engagements are infrequent, as she needs to be in bed by 10.30 p.m. She requires eight hours' sleep a night, which she usually achieves without taking sleeping pills.

There has been surprisingly little strain on Mary's marriage. Her writer husband is very understanding and leads his own busy life. Mary is also fortunate in that she has had no problems with her short-term memory—at least no more than others of her age. But she finds it necessary to limit her concentration to a maximum of an hour and a half. It is intense concentration for a limited period; quality rather than quantity.

Chapter seven

Coping with CFS

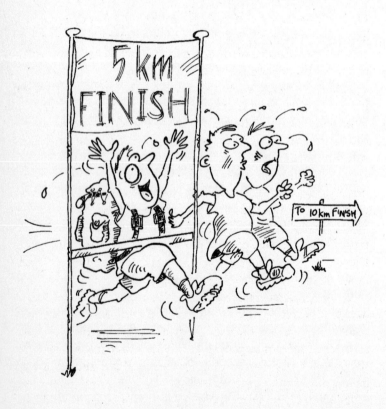

The principles of coping with CFS can be called the 'Four A' plan:

Accept the diagnosis.
Adapt your lifestyle.
Adjust your priorities.
Acknowledge your limits.

As with any chronic illness there are many factors that need to be considered regarding the long-term management of CFS. Unlike other conditions, coping with CFS must take into account the debilitating symptoms, the diversity of presentation and the controversial status of the disorder. These variables make it a difficult illness to manage and, above all, an illness that requires a different approach in different patients. There are, of course, many aspects of management that are common to all.

The way people comprehend the effects of CFS on their bodies will determine how well they adapt to the illness. Similarly, their health status prior to the illness is relevant to the way they cope with its diagnosis and its inevitably relapsing nature.

The earlier the diagnosis is made, the better the prognosis. This is so with most illnesses, but is especially significant with CFS. Because of its nature, a lengthy period of illness without an explanation can only serve to decrease the patient's self-confidence. It is also difficult for family and friends to offer support when they have no idea of the diagnosis or reason for the patient's condition.

Once the condition has been diagnosed, the patient must **accept** it and adjust his or her life accordingly. We cannot change the diagnosis, but we can **adapt** our lifestyle, our attitudes and our expectations. In a rather ironic way, the diagnosis of CFS often makes us re-evaluate our lives and develop new priorities as a result.

It can be difficult to change our priorities after a lifetime of setting goals and trying to achieve targets. To unlearn deeply ingrained ideals is almost impossible for some. We must at least **adjust** our priorities in accordance with our capabilities. If we improve as a result of this, then surely it is worth it. If our priorities are thought of as a sliding scale that can be adjusted, then we may be able to move back a little as we get better. But to return completely to a demanding self-imposed schedule is to invite a major relapse.

One of the first cases of CFS I came across was a real-estate salesman in his mid-twenties. His clinical progress was delayed considerably by his inability to adjust his priorities. The small amount of energy he had each day was totally dissipated by his hectic work schedule and irregular hours. It was only after he was admitted to hospital for extensive tests and complete rest that he began to realise the significance of his diagnosis.

The most important aspect of coping is learning to listen to your body. Your capabilities will vary from day to day, so there are no set rules. However, ignoring the limits of those capabilities at any time will invite an exacerbation of CFS. It is vital to **acknowledge** one's limits and remain within them.

It is very easy to become a victim of our ideals. In what has become a fast-lane society, it is sometimes a good thing to pull over and to consider where we are heading. During the first year of my illness I had no choice but to do so. With continued improvement, that course of action has been vindicated. I have also become aware of the many other ways I can contribute to society while also obtaining fulfilment. Other options (medical and social) continually present themselves and, if compatible with my capabilities, they can become a reality.

Management of CFS involves other people as well. Whether you are single or married, working or unemployed, retired or still at school, there are many others who are involved. Immediate family and close friends need to be aware of your special needs and limitations, as do teachers, work colleagues, and others in the community who are involved in providing health care and personal support services.

Despite an increased community awareness of the disorder, there is still a great deal of ignorance. In addition to coping with their illness, many patients have to contend with the rather controversial status of CFS. They find there are times when they become heartily sick of trying to explain what is a very complicated disorder to someone who knows little about it or thinks it is just about 'being constantly tired'. When the condition has stabilised and you are able to get out more, it will be helpful if you know how to handle such encounters. Most people do not deliberately set out to cause offence. Statements like 'Oh yes, I think I have it too. I am always tired!' usually reflect a lack of knowledge about the condition. The best way of dealing with it is to explain some of the many symptoms of CFS apart from the fatigue aspect. Some people are amazed to discover that muscle pain is a major symptom, or that balance disturbance and severe headaches are also quite common.

There will always be a few people who treat CFS as a 'condition of the mind'. They find it hard to appreciate that patients can look fit and healthy for a good deal of the time. In these situations it is best not to waste your time and energy. It is often much simpler to recommend they read about it!

Coping at home

Most CFS sufferers require an initial period at home after their condition has been diagnosed. This period is important in providing adequate rest and giving your body every chance to get over CFS as soon as possible. For many this involves lots of bed rest; their bedrooms become the centre of their lives.

How you cope with being restricted to bed depends largely on how you adapt to your surroundings. It is essential that you have within reach (literally) a telephone, a radio and a television, preferably with remote control. These items will keep you in touch with the outside world and enable you to communicate with family and friends.

An ample supply of reading material is also desirable. Being bed-bound is a good opportunity to catch up on books you may not have had time to read before. I found biographies especially satisfying as well as reference books that could be dipped into. Reading can aggravate eye muscle fatigue, which may limit the time spent reading, but it is nonetheless an enjoyable way of putting that time to good use.

Television can likewise be rewarding. Selective viewing makes one realise what an invaluable medium it is. There is often something worthwhile to watch at peak periods, and it is an ideal way of passive learning, especially when combined with video-recording.

Radio is ideal when you are too tired to read or watch television. Sadly, there is far too little quality radio, but, chosen carefully, it can be both entertaining and informative. Some of the best radio is community radio. In Melbourne this includes a station for the visually impaired, which I found very useful when reading a newspaper was not possible. Similar services for the print-handicapped exist in other capital cities in Australia, New Zealand and Canada. In the USA these facilities are not always available on open-band stations, but may be on an FM sub-carrier station or transmitted on the cable network. Similar radio facilities are available in the United Kingdom and in the larger cities of Europe.

Music lovers will have their own ways of filling in the time. Radio, CDs and tapes are an ideal solution. This was one of my salvations when ill. My involvement in preparing music and opera programs for Melbourne's only non-government classical music radio station, 3MBS-FM 103.5, was rewarding, therapeutic and very worthwhile.

There are some advantages in being bed-bound. The need for extra sleep in the first year of combating CFS made it very easy to nap during the day. You are also less tempted to do something that might prove exhausting. I mentioned earlier in Chapter 5 that gentle muscle exercises should be done in bed each day, and a suitable routine worked out. This is important to maintain muscle tone and aid the circulation.

There will be times when you are able to get out of bed and sit in a comfortable chair with your feet up for certain periods of the day. This allows a change of environment from the bedroom, and may be possible in the mornings for a little while after a bath or shower. As you improve, the time spent out of bed will increase; but to begin with it is very much a matter of trial and error.

It is important to adapt the home for the initial period when you will be at least home-bound, if not bed-bound. The muscular fatigue that prevents many from continuing in their normal occupation will also make home duties difficult. Home help is essential, and may involve getting outside help for the first time or extending your existing arrangements. Cleaning and vacuuming are impossible for most patients. Even making the bed may be a challenge for some. It is important to have a good working system whereby all domestic chores are taken care of. If you have a partner, then there will be a greater reliance on him or her. And children, if old enough, may need to accept more responsibility for certain chores if one parent is out of action.

You will soon work out which household tasks need to be delegated. Anything of a repetitive nature will cause myalgia, so many household and gardening activities will become impossible when CFS is at its worst. As frustrating as this may be, you must accept it, with the sure knowledge that things will get better.

Starting to mobilise

There are numerous aids available to help you cope with the disabling effects of CFS. If mobility is a problem due to feelings of imbalance, then strategically placed rails, especially in the bathroom, will help prevent accidents. Stairs are frequently a problem with CFS sufferers, so it may be worth considering a bedroom downstairs. Occasionally a walking frame or stick will help, especially if unsteadiness due to muscle weakness is a problem. In rare cases a wheelchair may be necessary when the symptoms are so severe as to prevent walking.

Some of the household aids available for sufferers of arthritis may also be useful in the home of the CFS sufferer. There are numerous gadgets available to help with such fundamental tasks as turning on a tap, opening a jar and chopping vegetables. Special non-slip mats in the shower and super-large towels make it easier to dry yourself after bathing.

Chairs should be comfortable and easy to get out of. Raised seats and adapted arms may be of use, as are adjustable recliners and footstools. Although it may sound unimportant, getting up from a chair frequently will soon cause fatigue, especially if you exert much effort in doing so.

Phone access is very important wherever you are. Extension phones or a mobile battery phone will enable you to answer calls without having to get up. This allows you to sit in the garden in fine weather, yet still keep in touch.

In the kitchen

In most modern kitchens, cupboards and appliances should be at an appropriate level. It is wise to avoid stretching too far or bending excessively. When I was at my worst one of my most dreaded tasks was unloading the dishwasher. This involved kneeling on the floor and taking out the plates, cups and cutlery in separate batches and placing them on the bench. After completing the task, still on my knees, I would then stand up slowly and proceed to put things away. Even to this day it is a chore I dislike, and yet the vast majority of dishwashers are installed below bench level.

Preparation of food should not be too great a problem. There are so many aids available, from food processors to electric can openers. Many cooking utensils have been specially designed to help prepare meals with minimal effort. Pre-prepared meals should be kept in the freezer for bad days. Casseroles are a good example of something that can be prepared in advance and frozen in individual serve sizes. Microwave ovens are great for heating such meals, as well as cooking vegetables quickly and effectively. A wok should be an essential part of every kitchen. It is easy to learn how to prepare a delicious Chinese meal with little effort. The ingredients can be prepared earlier and set aside, while the slices of meat or chicken are marinated. Steamed rice can be cooked in the microwave (or conventionally) and, when ready, the other ingredients stir-fried. Your meal is cooked in minutes and can be as good as anything you would order in a restaurant or spend hours preparing.

Pasta is another dish that is simple to cook. It can also be prepared in advance, as can the meat, chicken or fish. Sauces are easily prepared and can be frozen, and many can be bought from good supermarkets, ready to heat. Italian cuisine, like Asian dishes, adds variety to a diet and is fun to prepare. There is minimal effort involved.

Another dietary staple is home-made soup, based on chicken stock, fish stock or lamb shanks. This can be prepared when you are mobile, and is a great and traditional way of incorporating vegetables and either chicken or lamb into a nutritional broth that is easy to eat when you are having a bad day and are forced to remain in bed. Soups also freeze well and are a good standby during a relapse.

Shopping

Shopping for provisions can be organised without much difficulty. Usually a routine can be established whereby a family member, friend or neighbour will be happy to help. Some supermarkets will deliver. There will be times when you can manage yourself, with the assistance of a friend to drive you and help with any lifting. Certain items can be bought in bulk, and there should always be a supply of essential items for those times when you are not well enough to get out.

Driving

In the worst stages of CFS you should avoid driving a car. Any muscular exertion is bad, and even pulling on a handbrake after parking the car may cause painful myalgia and exhaustion. Getting into and out of a low car seat (as with most sports cars) frequently is also a problem. Most modern cars have automatic gears and power steering, and this is of course a huge help. Nevertheless, it is best to keep driving to a minimum and drive only for short distances until your condition has stabilised.

Parking a car can also be a difficult exercise. Merely turning and twisting the neck can bring on symptoms and, although this may sound exaggerated, the parking of a car is usually found to be far more difficult than driving it. Disability permits may help in this regard and are obtainable from your local council with a medical certificate from your doctor. This will allow you closer access to shopping centres and other facilities, and lessen the amount of walking. However, in the later, more stable phases of CFS you should forget the disability permit and make use of the walk. It is actually good for you!

Sleep disturbances

As discussed in Chapter 3, sleep disturbance is a common complaint in CFS sufferers. This problem is not helped by the fact that patients spend so much time in bed in the early stages of the illness. Napping during the day may upset normal sleep rhythms and make it difficult to get to sleep at night. Before resorting to pills it is worth noting some sleep hygiene rules, which are basically common sense and will benefit everyone.

- Relaxation techniques are an important aspect of preparing for sleep. The physical, mental and intellectual stimulation that occurs during the day can persist unless we make an effort to 'wind down' at night.
  - The hour before retiring should be spent reading a book, preferably non-fiction.
  - A warm bath, with herbal gel added, is recommended, especially if muscles are tense.
  - Practise slow, deep breathing, while lying or sitting down.
  - Allow the mind to wander (as opposed to meditation, where there is a central thought or 'mantra' on which to focus).
  - Gently flex and relax the various muscle groups to reach a state of total body relaxation.
- Avoid caffeine-containing drinks for four hours prior to sleeping. De-caffeinated tea and coffee are available and some herbal teas (e.g. camomile) are positively therapeutic. Alternatively, a glass of warm milk is usually helpful.
- Eliminate any physical pain or pressure. This may mean the use of an anti-inflammatory drug after dinner and/or an analgesic. Heavy bedding can be another source of pressure. A light continental quilt may be preferable to blankets, although the latter are adjusted more easily.
- Keep your bedroom comfortably warm but not over-heated. There should be a source of fresh air, and central heating should be switched off. Similarly, electric blankets should be used to warm the bed, but should be switched off once you are in bed.

A sleeping pill may be prescribed by your doctor if you are still having difficulty establishing a normal sleep pattern. These may only be necessary for a short period. Certainly, they should not be used as a substitute for the above steps.

An antidepressant may be considered appropriate in some CFS patients (as discussed in chapters 3 and 5). If this is given as a night-time dose it may have the beneficial advantage of inducing sleep.

Employment

One of the most serious consequences of any chronic illness is its effect on the patient's ability to work. Sufferers of CFS can usually look forward to an improvement in their condition, but the time factor is quite unpredictable. This makes planning for the future very difficult, and each case must be assessed individually.

In the early stages of CFS, most patients will be totally unable to work or study. All efforts must be directed at getting over this devastating period of disability. It is a mistake merely to reduce your workload and hope that you will somehow scrape through. I am convinced that, from the time CFS is diagnosed, your body must be given every opportunity to rest and recuperate.

Once you have started to improve and your condition stabilises, which in most cases will take at least a year, then a staged return to work may be possible. This will of course depend upon the conditions of your employment, and any provisions that are in place for sick leave and benefits. In any case, your doctor's opinion is of paramount importance and must be considered before you take any action regarding future work plans.

In my own case I found it extremely difficult to stop working completely. After many years of striving at school and university the inertia had continued. The thought of not getting up every morning and working a full day seemed almost incomprehensible. It was against my instincts. However, those months of enforced rest made me re-examine my own *raison d'être*.

If there is any doubt about your entitlements you should seek legal, and possibly union, advice on your individual situation. Financial assistance may be available in some cases, and in others there may even be a work-related component to the illness. You may also be entitled to disability income protection, or qualify for government-funded sickness benefits, depending on your financial situation.

Relationships

A chronic illness like CFS can strain relationships. Young sufferers may not always have the understanding of their peer groups, and may be affected at a crucial stage in their development. For this reason it is important that close friends/lovers/spouses/children be fully educated about CFS and its possible ramifications.

Marriages can be put at risk despite partners' best intentions. Some partners have difficulty in coping with the long-term disability of a spouse. The increased demands upon the well partner can be very wearing over time. Sexual relationships will almost certainly be affected. The physical aspects of sex depend on a certain degree of fitness, both physical and mental. The muscle pains and total exhaustion of CFS can make sex difficult, and for this reason allowances should be made by both partners. Further negative influences on libido can occur if the patient is depressed by the illness, or as a side-effect of some antidepressants used to treat such a patient. Should these medications be necessary, the possible side-effects should always be discussed with your doctor.

Holidays

When CFS is at its worst the idea of a holiday is out of the question. However, when the illness has stabilised and you are aware of your limitations it may be possible to arrange a holiday with friends or family members. It is best not to go too far afield for a number of reasons.

Crossing time zones can be taxing even for those who are well. Jet lag is a common problem, but it is much worse in the CFS sufferer. Even with copious amounts of fluid, no alcohol and lots of rest at both ends, a long flight can still bring on a relapse in CFS patients. For this reason, holidays should be relatively simple. Travelling by car, or by plane for a short trip only is generally safe. A change of environment and climate can work wonders, but you don't have to travel halfway around the world.

There are other reasons why long trips should be postponed until your condition has stabilised. Carrying luggage, standing in airport queues, and checking in and out of different venues can be exhausting for anyone. With CFS it can be a nightmare and can precipitate a relapse, undoing the potential good of any holiday. So, until you are much better, keep holiday plans simple and enjoy them all the more.

Vaccinations

From the outset, I must say that I thoroughly endorse all the usual childhood vaccinations. There is no good reason why a child should have to suffer pertussis (whooping cough), poliomyelitis, diphtheria, measles and tetanus—all of which can be life-threatening—merely because these is a very small chance of a side-effect and because their parents were misguided enough to deny them protection.

In the case of CFS it is possible that vaccinations may precipitate a relapse in some patients. Even so, it is still my belief that a child with CFS should be vaccinated at a suitable time. This could be during a remission in their illness, and at a time when they have ample opportunity to rest following the vaccination—perhaps during holiday time.

In older patients, a similar approach should be taken. Any possible exacerbation in their symptoms should be weighed up against the very real danger they face if they remain unprotected. For example, an avid gardener would be foolish to refuse a tetanus booster on the grounds that it may cause a flare-up in his CFS symptoms. Other things might too, but meanwhile he could die of tetanus!

In the case of overseas travel vaccinations, there may be a choice. Cholera and typhoid are not usually necessary, and typhoid, especially, can cause a nasty reaction, even in the healthy person. On the other hand, if you are visiting a country where yellow fever is endemic you must be vaccinated. Have the shots well in advance when you can allow yourself ample rest following the vaccination.

Other instances of vaccinations need to be considered on an individual basis. Most CFS sufferers would be wise to avoid having the annual influenza vaccinations unless they are especially at risk. They are of limited protection in terms of the huge number of respiratory viruses circulating in a normal community in winter. There are other precautions you can take (sensible warm clothing, vitamin C, and, where possible, avoiding contact with flu sufferers).

On the other hand, occupational risks may make it wise to be vaccinated, despite having had CFS. Nurses and doctors who come into contact with blood and serum products should be protected against hepatitis B. It is a severe enough illness in its own right (with the potential to cause liver damage) to justify this prophylactic approach. It you are well enough to work, you should be able to withstand the vaccination; but have it at a suitable time when you can rest adequately afterwards.

CFS and pregnancy

CFS and pregnancy are not incompatible. Many patients with CFS are women of child-bearing age who may well have delayed getting pregnant because of their illness. Others have gone ahead and had a family despite ill health. And some have become pregnant accidentally while suffering CFS.

Obviously this is a difficult decision. Even if you have had CFS and largely recovered from it, getting pregnant may precipitate a relapse. Yet, strangely, in many patients there is a marked improvement in CFS symptoms during the course of pregnancy. This is presumably due to the hormone changes that occur at this time.

We have known for many years that the incidence of abnormalities in pregnancy rises with the age of the mother. For those over the age of 40 the risks become very significant indeed. So there is already a certain limit to how long you should wait before trying to conceive. There does not appear to be an increase in the rate of miscarriages in CFS patients.

As a general rule it is best to consider pregnancy only if your condition has greatly improved and your CFS has been stable for at least a year. Even then you should discuss the matter with your doctor first, and be aware of the possible complications. For most women the challenge will come at the end of the pregnancy. It is during labour, in particular, that their strength will be tested and their CFS may let them down.

The antenatal management of a patient with CFS does not differ greatly from the normal patient. The same screening tests are performed and you visit your doctor regularly throughout the pregnancy. Blood pressure, urine tests and weight gain are all documented; an ultrasound is routinely performed to check for abnormalities in your baby's development.

Ironically, CFS patients often cope better with the aches and pains of pregnancy than other would-be mums. They have stated that the discomfort of pregnancy is nowhere near as bad as the painful aches of their CFS at its worst. They seem better prepared to cope with discomfort and are more than ready to put up with it when they consider the end result.

Despite the frequent improvement in their CFS during pregnancy, these patients still need ample rest. An unfortunate minority appears to suffer a worsening of symptoms during pregnancy. These women need to conserve their strength and to prepare for the enormous demands placed upon them during labour and in the immediate post-natal period, when practical matters such as breastfeeding and looking after babies will be of prime importance.

CFS and labour

Although there has been no detailed research, preliminary studies suggest that approximately half of all CFS patients who become pregnant are prone to some complication— either during pregnancy or during labour—as a result of their illness. Epidural anaesthesia and the use of forceps are thought to be more likely as a result of exhaustion during labour and a loss of muscle strength. It is also likely that CFS patients need more rest late in their pregnancy, as well as after labour.

The incidence of Caesarean section is thought to be higher in CFS patients. This is presumably due to exhaustion during labour, as well as any other indications that may exist for a surgical delivery. If the labour has been long and exhausting there is also likely to be a greater need for pain-relieving injections.

The post-partum challenge

It is important that a CFS patient is not discharged too soon after giving birth. She will need extra rest after what is frequently an exhausting labour which may, in some cases, cause an exacerbation of her illness. In addition, she will need to learn how to breastfeed and care for the new baby. This period of after-care hospitalisation is an opportunity to get accustomed to this exciting new aspect of her life.

Although most women experience an improvement in their CFS symptoms during pregnancy, the post-partum period frequently sees a return to their former pattern. They certainly need more rest after labour than the normal patient, and this pattern continues after their discharge. All the trials and joys of being a new mother are exaggerated for the CFS patient, and it is important that the home situation is prepared for the extra demands and stresses put on her.

The majority of CFS mothers will have mild to moderate symptoms. These will increase with exercise and activity and, as a result, these women will experience some degree of decreased activity or functioning. Most will be unable to perform tasks requiring physical labour, but the majority will be able to perform light tasks and care for their children.

Most new mothers with CFS will concentrate their efforts on their baby. Feeding is a special priority and most will start by putting their baby on the breast. They face the same problems as every other new mother, and some will have to wean the baby sooner than they would have liked if there is insufficient breastmilk production, if the baby has a sucking problem, if mastitis is present, or if any of the symptoms of CFS start to predominate.

There are obvious advantages in bottle-feeding infants. If there is help at home to wash bottles and prepare feeds it will allow a frequently exhausted CFS mother more time to rest. Husbands, grandparents and others can feed the baby, as well as help with other tasks such as bathing the baby and changing nappies. The advantages of breastfeeding for baby's immune system and emotional well-being are sometimes over-emphasised, and no mother should feel she has failed if her baby has to be weaned earlier than planned, for whatever reason.

The arrival of a new baby is an occasion to celebrate. I know of no CFS patient who has regretted having a child, even if it has been a difficult pregnancy and there have been other post-natal problems. With proper planning, family support and due consideration from obstetric staff, it is manageable in all but the most severe cases of CFS.

It is in this situation that the 'Four A' plan is especially relevant. Being realistic and **accepting** your condition will mean you should be aware of the potential problems that lie ahead. **Adapting** your lifestyle and acknowledging the additional limitations imposed by pregnancy will help you to prepare. **Adjusting** your priorities and putting the needs of the baby uppermost are obviously vital. **Acknowledging** your limits will also ensure that you accept the assistance of family, friends and the community in bringing a new life into this world in the most favourable of environments.

CFS and the school-age child

The incidence of CFS in children is much lower than among adults, but it has been increasingly recognised in recent years. School-age children can be affected and there is not much difference in the symptomatology to adult sufferers. However, the treatment differs in some respects and the long-term implications can be quite serious if it is badly managed.

The predominant symptoms in children are fatigue, myalgia and sleep disturbances. The muscle involvement is particularly marked, and in some cases can lead to muscle wasting and even contractures (fixed muscle resistance and related joint deformity). Fatigue is another prominent complaint and, unfortunately, one that can be misinterpreted by parents and teachers alike. The resultant sleep disturbance can lead to a sleep reversal pattern where the child sleeps by day and is awake at night.

In some cases of childhood CFS there is a known viral infection at the start. As a result, the condition has sometimes been misdiagnosed as 'post-viral debility'. Although this may be partly correct, it fails to take into account the more insidious abnormalities of the immune system. There has been a fundamental overstimulation of the immune reaction and an excess production of cytokines, or chemicals that circulate in high concentration for a much longer period than any normal post-viral malaise.

Treatment in children involves alternating rest with a graduated exercise program. However, it is important that the child's progress is carefully monitored, because too much rest will lead to muscle atrophy and long-term problems with muscle contractures, bone thinning and growth disturbances. The ideal management appears to be a carefully balanced program of rest, alternating with graded exercises or activity that will not produce a relapse. There is much less reason to use medication in children. Paracetamol may be necessary for muscle pain, but anti-inflammatory and antidepressant drugs are not usually indicated. There is a greater need for counselling in children because of their difficulty in coming to terms with a chronic illness that causes disruption to their progress at school, keeps them at home away from friends, and isolates them from the world at a most important stage of their development.

The long-term effects of CFS on a child will depend on how the illness is managed. There should be a team approach, with parents, teachers, the family doctor and a child psychologist meeting to determine how best to guide the patient. In anticipation of a prolonged recovery, it would also be advisable for the GP to involve a paediatrician who is familiar with CFS and its potentially damaging sequelae.

The effects of CFS on a child's academic achievements will depend upon how successful the 'team effort' has been. Quite obviously, the longer the absence from school, the more serious will be the effect. However, there is little point in the child returning prematurely, only to suffer a relapse and be back in bed, feeling worse than ever. The provision of home tutorials and perhaps some personal coaching is ideal and enables the child to keep up academically. Yet, it is important to set a realistic pace, determined by the child's clinical progress.

Weight loss can be another problem in children with CFS.

Unlike adult patients, who tend to eat 'for energy' and don't always burn up the calories by their relative inactivity, a sick child tends not to eat. School-age children sometimes go through periods of 'fad' diets, which are often unbalanced. If there is added emotional stress, like a chronic illness, their bodies can react by becoming anorexic. This must be guarded against, because a suitable diet, along with rest and lifestyle adaptation, is one of the most important aspects of treatment.

The careful balance of rest and graded activity will eventually result in improvement. However, as with adults, a premature return to normal activities will exacerbate the illness. This applies to both physical and mental endeavours, and is especially relevant to school-age children who may not always be the best judges of how much they can do. When the child is ready to return to school it should be on a part-time basis to begin with, and a strictly limited amount of homework, exercise, and social activity should leave adequate time for rest.

Children sometimes have great difficulty in coping with the isolation of a long-term illness. Being forced out of mainstream school activities can be a frightening experience, coming at a very vulnerable stage of their development. It is for this reason that emotional counselling is an important part of their treatment.

Most children with CFS make a complete recovery. When the diagnosis is made early and there is an initial period of complete rest, combined with a good diet as discussed in Chapter 5, the grounds are laid for positive progress. With the introduction of the balanced activity program and the team approach, the prognosis should be very promising.

Some children's progress at school will be minimally affected. Others may need to repeat a year. With adequate communication between parents, doctor, teachers and counsellor, the disruption to a child's education should be minimised.

Conclusion

CFS is a diverse illness of uncertain aetiology and indeterminate duration. It is much more complex than its name would imply, both in its symptomatology and its ramifications. The aetiology probably involves many factors, resulting in an abnormality or overreaction of the immune system.

For most patients, the diagnosis of CFS is both a relief and a challenge. It is reassuring to have an explanation for such debilitating symptoms, and yet the implications are far-reaching. The need to pace yourself is one of the most important aspects of its management.

The ability to cope with CFS will depend on your ability to adapt to the illness. The drastic limitations imposed by this condition make you re-evaluate life and appreciate things previously taken for granted. In my own case, there have been many positive aspects to CFS, one of which has been the chance to broaden my interests.

Above all, there is cause to be optimistic. The majority of CFS patients do get better. It may take years, but, with continuing self-discipline and a modified lifestyle, the lights at the end of the tunnel are shining as brightly as ever.

Useful organisations

Various CFS support groups exist in most countries. These are usually in the larger cities and are often run by volunteers, with input from professionals with an interest in the condition. Most aspects of the illness are dealt with, and these societies are valuable in educating the wider community about CFS through lectures with guest speakers and regular publications. As well as providing information to patients about the various services available, they offer counselling to patients and their families, and liaise with the media to project a more positive and realistic image of CFS.

Australia
New South Wales
   ME/CFS Society of New South Wales Inc.
   Royal South Sydney Community Health Complex
   Joynton Avenue
   Zetland NSW 2017
   Tel: 02 9439 6026
   NSW country areas: 1300 659 026 (toll-free)
   Fax: 02 9382 8160
   Email: mesoc@zip.com.au
   Web: http://www.zip.com.au/~mesoc

Australian Capital Territory
ACT ME/CFS Society Inc.
C/- SHOUT Office
PO Box 717
Mawson ACT 2607

Collett Place
Pearce ACT 2607
Tel: 02 6290 1984
Fax: 02 6286 4475
Email: shout@cybermac.com.au
Web: http://spirit.net.au/~masmith/

Victoria and Tasmania
ME/CFS Society of Victoria Inc.
23 Livingstone Close
Burwood VIC 3125
Tel: 03 9888 8798
Fax: 03 9888 8991
Email: mecfs@vicnet.net.au
Web: http://www.vicnet.net.au/~mecfs

South Australia
ME/CFS Society of South Australia Inc.
GPO Box 383
Adelaide SA 5001

195 Gilles Street
Adelaide SA 5000
Tel: 08 8223 7722
Fax: 08 8227 0922
Email: cfs_soc_sa@freemail.com.au
Web: http://sacfs.tsx.org

Queensland
ME/CFS Society of Queensland Inc.
PO Box 938
Fortitude Valley QLD 4006

134 St Paul's Terrace
Spring Hill QLD 4000
Tel: 07 3832 9744
Fax: 07 3832 9755

Western Australia
ME/CFS Society of Western Australia Inc.
C/- WISH
PO Box 8140
Perth Business Centre WA 6849
Tel: 08 9228 4488
Fax: 08 9228 4490

New Zealand
ANZMES Society
PO Box 36 307
Northcote
Auckland
NEW ZEALAND
Tel: 09 480 7356
Web: http://www.anzmes.org

United Kingdom
The ME Association was established in 1976 and has a network
of self-help groups throughout the United Kingdom. Further
details may be obtained by contacting:
ME Association of Great Britain
4 Corringham Road
Stanford-le-Hope
Essex
UNITED KINGDOM SS17 0AH
Tel: 01375 642 466
Fax: 01375 360 256
Web: www.meassociation.org.uk

Action for ME
PO Box 1302
Wells
Somerset BA 51YE
England
Tel: 01749 670 799
Fax: 01749 672 561
Web: www.afme.org.uk

ME Association, Scotland Region
52 St Enoch Square
Glasgow G1 4AA, Scotland
Tel: 0141 204 3822

Irish ME Support Group
PO Box 3075
Dublin 2
Ireland
Tel: 01235 0965

ME Association, Northern Ireland Region
Bryson House
28 Bedford St, Belfast
BT2 7FE
Tel/Fax: 01232 439 831

Europe

Danish ME/CFS Organisation
Radhustorvet 1,2
DK-3520 Farum
Denmark
Tel: 45 44 95 97 00
Fax: 45 44 95 97 74

CFS/CFIDS Self Help Group, Germany
Lubener Weg 3
D-53119 Bonn
Germany

CFS Association, Italy
Segreteria: Via Moimacco 20
33100 Udine
Italy

USA
There are many support networks throughout the USA. The various States have their own listings. Further information may be obtained by contacting:
The CFIDS Association of America
PO Box 220398
Charlotte NC 28222-0398
USA

Tel: 704 362 2343
Fax: 704 365 9755
Email: info@cfids.org
Web: http://www.cfids.org

The National CFIDS Foundation, Inc.
103 Aletha Road
Needham, MA 02492-3931
USA
Tel: 781 449 3535
Fax: 781 449 8606

CFIDS and Fibromyalgia Health Resource, California
1187 Coast Village Road, Suite 1-280
Santa Barbara, CA 93108-2794
Tel: 800 366 6056
Fax: 805 965 0042

CFS Crisis Centre, New York
27 W. 20th Street, Suite 703
New York, NY 10011
USA
Tel: 212 691 4800

Canada

ME Association of Canada
Suite 4200, 246 Queen Street
Ottawa
Ontario
CANADA K1P5E4
Tel: 613 563 1565
Fax: 613 567 0614
Email: info@mecan.ca
Web: http://www.mecan.ca

South Africa

ME Association of South Africa
PO Box 1802
Umhlanga Rocks 4320
Natal
SOUTH AFRICA

Glossary

anaemia   a reduction in the number of red blood cells and/or the amount of haemoglobin within them

antibody   a serum globulin synthesised in lymphoid tissue in response to antigenic stimulation

antigen   a (usually) protein-containing substance which, when foreign to the circulation, will stimulate the formation of a specific antibody

atrophy   shrinking in size (or wasting) of body tissue

autoimmune disease   an altered immune response where the body produces a reaction to its own tissue

bradycardia   decreased heart rate

carcinogen   a cancer-causing substance

cognitive dysfunction   disturbed concentration, short-term memory and word-finding ability

cortisol   a hormone produced by the cortex of the adrenal gland with physiological effects similar to cortisone

cytokine   a body chemical manufactured or activated by the immune system in response to infection, and produced in excessive amounts in CFS

dysphagia   difficulty in swallowing

dystonia   disordered muscle tone

epidemiology   the study of the incidence and distribution of a disorder within a community

Epstein-Barr virus (EBV)   a member of the herpes group of viruses, known to be one of the causes of infectious mononucleosis (glandular fever)

erythrocyte   red blood cell

erythrocyte sedimentation rate (ESR)   the speed at which erythrocytes agglutinate and sediment; it is measured in the laboratory, and is raised in a range of illnesses, especially inflammatory conditions, but is non-specific as a test

extrasystole   a premature or extra heart beat, independent of the normal rhythm

fibromyalgia   musculoskeletal pain (generalised or regional) and abnormal areas of soft-tissue tenderness

glossitis   inflammation of the tongue

granulocytosis   an abnormally large number of granulo- cytes, i.e. leucocytes or white blood cells containing neutrophil, basophil or eosinophil granules in the cytoplasm of the cell

haemoglobin   the oxygen-carrying pigment of the red blood cell

hyperacusis   abnormal acuteness of hearing or a painful sensation to sounds

hyperaesthesia   increased skin sensitivity

hypercalcaemia   an excess of calcium in the blood

hypersomnia   an abnormally increased sleep requirement

hyper- or hypotension   raised or lowered blood pressure

hypokalaemia   lowered level of potassium in the blood

immunoglobulin   a protein in the serum that has the task of an antibody (e.g. in neutralising a virus)

infectious mononucleosis   glandular fever

ischaemia   deficiency of blood supply to part of the body, e.g. myocardinal ischaemia (reduced blood flow to the heart muscle)

ketones   a carbonyl-containing substance that may be found in urine in poorly controlled diabetics, in cases of prolonged fasting or vomiting, or where the diet has been very high in fats and low in carbohydrates

leucocyte white blood cell

leucocytosis an increased number of white blood cells

liver function test (LFT) a measure in the blood of specific enzymes, raised levels of which can indicate inflammation or other pathology of the liver

lymphocyte a variety of white blood cell that arises in the lymph glands

lymphadenopathy diseased lymph nodes which may be enlarged or palpable, indicating involvement in an infectious or malignant process

lymphocytosis a raised number of lymphocytes, commonly found in the early stages of an infection

macrocytic refers to a condition where the red blood cells are larger than usual

macrophage a 'scavenger' cell that takes up infected cells and invading organisms, part of the network of events that leads to the production of antibodies

magnetic resonance imaging (MRI) a sensitive imaging test measuring magnetic resonance of bodily tissues by charting electromagnetic radiation being given off from the tissues; especially useful in neurological conditions

metastatic the transfer of disease (usually malignancies) from one organ or tissue to another

myelin a fatty type of substance forming a sheath around certain nerve fibres

myalgia painful muscles

neoplasm a malignant tumour

nystagmus an involuntary rapid movement of the eyeballs

oesophageal spasm involuntary spasm of part of the muscular wall of the oesophagus, causing localised stricture

osteoporosis the thinning of bone due to loss of calcium

palpitations unduly rapid action of the heart that is felt by the patient

paraesthesia abnormal skin sensation

perfusion the passage of fluid (e.g. blood) through the vessels of an organ or tissue

photophobia   intolerance to bright light

platelet   a circular or oval cell concerned with coagulation of the blood, and contraction of the blood clot; an intrinsic part of haemostasis and thrombosis

proctalgia fugax   pain in the rectum due to involuntary muscle spasm

rapid eye movement (REM) sleep   the light phase of sleep during which dreams occur

Raynaud's phenomenon   intermittent attacks of pallor or cyanosis of the extremities, especially fingers and toes, caused by an over-sensitive reaction to cold

single photon emission computed tomography (SPECT) a sensitive test of perfusion where the patient is given radioactive isotopes, and the radiation emitted can be used to measure blood flow in various parts of the brain

stomatitis   inflammation of the oral mucosa (lining of the mouth)

syncope   a temporary loss of consciousness and strength, as in a faint

tachycardia   increased heart rate

tinnitus   an abnormal noise in the ears, e.g. ringing, buzzing or whistling

thyroid function test (TFT)   a measure in the blood of the level of thyroid hormones, used to exclude under- or over-activity of the thyroid gland

urea and electrolytes (U&E)   an increase in the level of urea in the blood indicates reduced kidney function; and the electrolytes (body salts) are usually measured at the same time

vertigo   a sensation as if the external world were revolving around the patient (objective v.) or as if the patient were revolving in space (subjective v.)

vesicular   a blistery type of lesion (typically rash)

Bibliography

Bates D.W., Buchwald D., Lee J., Koth P. et al., 'Clinical
Test Findings in Patients with Chronic Fatigue Syndrome', *Archives of Internal Medicine*, 1995, 155,
97–103.

Behan P.O. and Barham A.M.O., 'Clinical Spectrum of
Post-viral Fatigue Syndrome', *British Medical Bulletin*,
1991, 47, 4, 793–808.

Behan P.O., Chaudhuri A., Majeed T. and Dinan T.,
'Chronic Fatigue Syndrome: A Disorder of Central
Cholinergic Transmission', *Journal of Chronic Fatigue
Syndrome*, 1997, 3(1), 3–15.

Bell D.S., *The Doctor's Guide to Chronic Fatigue Syndrome*, 1993, Addison-Wesley Publishing Company,
USA. **Note:** The author has extensively researched
chronic fatigue syndrome (known as Chronic Fatigue/
Immune Dysfunction Syndrome or CFIDS in the USA).
He combines his thorough knowledge with considerable
clinical experience of the illness to produce an account
that is concise, compassionate, and up-to-date.

Bell D.S., 'Chronic Fatigue Update', *Postgraduate
Medicine*, 1994, Vol. 96/1, 73–81.

Bon-Holaigah I., Rowe P.C., Kan J. and Calkins H., 'The relationship Between Neurally Mediated Hypotension and the Chronic Fatigue Syndrome', *Journal of the American Medical Association,* 1995, 274, 961–67.

Buchwald D. et al., 'A Chronic Illness Characterised by Fatigue, Neurologic and Immunologic Disorders and Active Human Herpesvirus Type 6 Infection', *Annals of Internal Medicine,* 1992, 116, 103–13.

Butler S. et al., 'Cognitive Behavior Therapy in the Chronic Fatigue Syndrome', *Journal of Neurology, Neurosurgery and Psychiatry,* 1991, 54, 153–58.

Caliguri M. et al., 'Phenotypic and Functional Deficiencies of Natural Killer Cells in Patients with Chronic Fatigue Syndrome', *Journal of Immunology,* 1987, 139, 3306–13.

Cheney P., 'Glutathione Deficiency in M.E./C.F.S. Patients' *Emerge: Journal of M.E./Chronic Fatigue Syndrome Society of Victoria Inc.,* Summer 1999. Originally published in *The National Forum,* Summer 1999, Vol. 3, No. 1.

Dunstan R.H., Donohoe M., Taylor W., Roberts T.K. et al., 'A Preliminary Investigation of Chlorinated Hydrocarbons and Chronic Fatigue Syndrome', *Medical Journal of Australia,* 18 Sept. 1995, 294–97.

Field E.J., 'Darwin's Illness', *Lancet,* 1990, 336, 826.

Fukuda K., Straus S.E., Hickie I., Sharpe M.C. et al., 'The Chronic Fatigue Syndrome: A Comprehensive Approach to its Definition and Study', *Annals of Internal Medicine,* 1994, 121, 953–59.

Gupta S. et al., 'A Comprehensive Immunological Analysis in Chronic Fatigue Syndrome', *Scandinavian Journal of Immunology,* 1991, 33, 319–27.

Heffez D., 'Can Spinal Surgery Really Help?', *Emerge: Journal of M.E./Chronic Fatigue Syndrome Society of Victoria Inc.,* Autumn 2000. Originally published in *CFIDS Chronicle,* 1999, Vol. 12, No. 6.

Hickie I. et al., 'The Psychiatric Status of Patients with the

Chronic Fatigue Syndrome', *British Journal of Psychiatry*, 1990, 156, 534–40.

Hinds G.M.E. and McCluskey D.R., 'A Retrospective Study of the Chronic Fatigue Syndrome', *Proceedings of the Royal College of Physicians, Edinburgh*, 1993, 23, 10–14.

Kendell R., 'Chronic Fatigue, Viruses and Depression', *Lancet*, 1991, 337, 160–63.

Klimas, N.G. et al., 'Immunological Abnormalities in Chronic Fatigue Syndrome', *Journal of Clinical Microbiology*, 1990, 28, 1403–10.

Komaroff A., 'The Komaroff Lecture', First World Congress on CFS and Related Disorders, Brussels, 9 Nov. 1995, in *Emerge: Journal of M.E./Chronic Fatigue Syndrome Society of Victoria Inc.*, June 1996, 32–5. Originally published in *Perspectives*, M.E. Association (UK), March 1996.

Lask B. and Dillon M.J. 'Postviral Fatigue Syndrome', *Archives of Disease in Childhood*, 1990, 65, 1198.

Lloyd A., 'An International Perspective on CFS Research', *Emerge: Journal of General Practice*, 1991, 91, 4, 339–42.

Lloyd A., Hickie I. and Wakerfield D., 'Immunological Abnormalities in Chronic Fatigue Syndrome', *Medical Journal of Australia*, 1990, 152, 51–2.

Lloyd A.R., 'Muscle and Brain: Chronic Fatigue Syndrome', *Medical Journal of Australia*, 1990, 153, 530–34.

Lloyd A.R. et al., 'What Is Myalgic Encephalomyelitis?', *Lancet*, 1988, 1, 1286–87.

Lloyd A.R. et al., 'Prevalence of Chronic Fatigue Syndrome in an Australian Population', *Medical Journal of Australia*, 1990, 153, 522–28.

Lloyd A.R. et al., 'Muscle Performance, Voluntary Activation, Twitch Properties and Perceived Effort in Normal Subjects and Patients with Chronic Fatigue Syndrome', *Brain*, 1991, 114, 85–9.

Lynch S. et al., 'Antidepressant Therapy in the Chronic Fatigue Syndrome', *British Journal of General Practice*, 1991, 91, 4, 339–42.

Marmion B., 'Post Q Fever Fatigue', *Lancet*, 6 April 1996.

McGregor N.R., Dunstan R.H., Roberts T.K. et al, 'Preliminary Determination of a Molecular Basis to Chronic Fatigue Syndrome', *Biochemical and Molecular Medicine*, 1996, 51, 73–80.

McGregor N.R., Dunstan R.H., Zerbes M., Roberts T.K. et al., 'Preliminary Determination of the Association between Symptom Expression and Urinary Metabolites in Subjects with Chronic Fatigue Syndrome', *Biochemical and Molecular Medicine*, 1996, 58, 85–92.

Morriss R.K., Weardon A.J. and Battersby L., 'The Relation of Sleep Difficulties to Fatigue, Mood and Disability in Chronic Fatigue Syndrome', *Journal of Psychosomatic Research*, 1997, 42(6), 597–605.

Oldmeadow M., 'The Management of Chronic Fatigue Syndrome', *Emerge: Journal of M.E./Chronic Fatigue Syndrome Society of Victoria Inc.*, June 1995, 24–6.

Parker S., Brukner P. and Rosier M., 'Chronic Fatigue Syndrome and the Athlete', *Sports Medicine, Training and Rehabilitation*, 1996, 6, 269–78.

Pearn J.H., 'Chronic Fatigue Syndrome: Chronic Ciguatera Poisoning as a Differential Diagnosis', *Medical Journal of Australia*, 17 March 1997, Vol. 166, 309–10.

Rowe P.C., Bon-Holaigah I., Kan J.S. and Calkins H., 'Is Neurally Mediated Hypotension an Unrecognised Cause of Chronic Fatigue?', *Lancet*, 1995, 345, 623–24.

Sharpe M. et al., 'Follow-up of Patients Presenting with Fatigue to an Infectious Disease Clinic', *British Medical Journal*, 1992, 305, 147–52.

Shepherd C., *Living with M.E.*, Second edition 1992, Cedar Books, UK. **Note:** A well-written, thoroughly researched and most comprehensive guide to all aspects of chronic fatigue syndrome (known as ME or myalgic encephalomyelitis in the United Kingdom). The author suffered the illness for years and writes from a sympathetic and authoritative viewpoint. An excellent book.

Straus S.E. et al., 'Acyclovir Treatment of Chronic Fatigue Syndrome; Lack of Efficacy in a Placebo-controlled Trial', *New England Journal of Medicine*, 1988, 26, 1692–98.

Twombly R., 'The Trouble with M.E.', *New Scientist*, 14 May 1994, 21–3.

Vercoulen J.H.M.M., Swanick C.M.A., Zitman F.G. et al., 'Randomised, Double-blind, Placebo-controlled Study of Fluoxetine in Chronic Fatigue Syndrome', *Lancet*, 1996, 347, 858–61.

Vollmer-Conna U., Hickie I., Hadzi-Parlovic D., Tymms K., Wakefield D., Dwyer J. and Lloyd A., 'Intravenous Immunoglobulin is Ineffective in the Treatment of Patients with Chronic Fatigue Syndrome', *American Journal of Medicine*, 1997, 103, 38–43.

Von Mikecz A. et al., 'High Frequencies of Autoantibodies to Insoluble Cellular Antigens in Patients with Chronic Fatigue Syndrome', *Arthritis and Rheumatism*, 1997, 40(2), 295–305.

Wakefield D., Lloyd A. and Hickie I., 'Chronic Fatigue Syndrome: Diagnosis and Treatment', *General Practitioner*, 23 March–5 April 1994, 5–6.

Wilson A. et al., 'Longitudinal Study of Outcome of Chronic Fatigue Syndrome', *British Medical Journal*, 1994, 308, 756–59.

Woodward R.V., Broom D.H. and Legge D.G., 'Diagnosis in Chronic Illness: Disabling or Enabling: the Case of Chronic Fatigue Syndrome', *Journal of the Royal Society of Medicine*, June 1995, Vol. 88, 325–29.

Index